# Diabetes
## and the
## Hypoglycemic
## Syndrome

Facts, Findings and Natural Treatments

Recipe Section

Calvin L. Thrash, M.D., MPH

Agatha M. Thrash, M.D., FACP

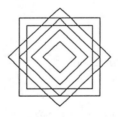

NEWLIFESTYLE BOOKS
SEALE, AL 36875

3

Diabetes and the Hypoglycemic Syndrome
Facts, Findings and Natural Treatments
By Calvin L. Thrash, M.D., MPH and
Agatha M. Thrash, M.D., FACP

A NewLifestyle Book / May, 1993

PRINTED IN THE UNITED STATES OF AMERICA
By Rose Printing, Tallahassee, FL

Original Printing, December, 1993
500 copies
Revised, March, 1994
Second Printing, November, 1994
2500 copies
Third Printing, January, 1996
2500 copies
Fourth Printing, June, 1997
2500 copies
Fifth Printing, April, 1999
5000 copies

ISBN: 0-942658-11-6

# Contents

# *Appreciation*

---

All wisdom is the result of bits of knowledge gleaned from many different sources. Similarly, all books result from knowledge acquired at many different times and from multiple people. We wish to thank our

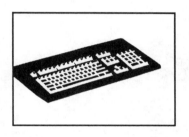

longtime friend and co-worker, Phylis Austin, for her great resourcefulness in providing just the right information at the right time.

The art work and technical assistance for this book were provided by our son, Cal Thrash, III, who has always been of good cheer and loving encouragement. Don Miller deserves our appreciation for providing advice and drawing graphs.

But the lion's share of work fell on the shoulders of our treasured editorial assistant, Donna Levine. Her tireless computer efforts and constant urging combined to organize and complete the book.

We can only say: Thank you. It has been a joy to work with each of you. We pray this book will be a blessing to many and your efforts will be repaid, knowing you have helped those who suffer with the common metabolic problems of diabetes and hypoglycemia, to achieve improvements in health.

# *Preface*

For generations, both the diagnosis and treatment of diabetes and the hypoglycemic syndrome, have been bogged down in a quagmire of error, ignorance and superstition, sometimes even by those who believe and claim to be experts in these areas.

Those who pioneered in researching diabetes and 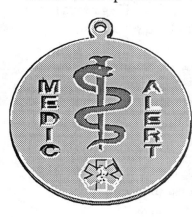 hypoglycemia presented theories about these two diseases that, at first, appeared logical and without fault. Because of the supposed correctness of these theories, and the reverence which students have given the researchers, honest errors have been perpetuated. Since students tend to shape their philosophies and practices upon the suppositions of their teachers, with something akin to superstitious zeal, little research was done until recently, that would correct the errors.

If we are to become freed from errors, the strict observance of scientific principles must be applied to all of our observations, or cherished myths will be perpetuated. It is not wrong to entertain theories based on intuition or feeling before facts are accumulated. But if it can be seen that diagnosis is lagging years behind the actual presence of a disease or disability, and that the current treatment is not producing desired results, there must be a change in theory and principle. Honesty then demands that we forfeit our cherished theories, face our fears of the unknown and try a different method. To know, or to seek to learn what we do not know, is of itself a higher form of knowledge.

## *Control Devices for Blood Sugar*

Our Heavenly Father did not want us to be inconvenienced by anything, especially not pain and discomfort. He designed thousands upon thousands of simple and complex mechanisms in the body, to enable us to perform the ordinary bodily functions with a minimum of effort and attention. Since the blood sugar level helps us in so many areas, including the control of temperament, maintaining cheerfulness and mental concentration, developing ambition, and a hundred other mental, physical and emotional functions, He gave us not one, but six major control devices for blood sugar:

1. The gastrointestinal tract, with precise control of stomach emptying and the exact concentration of nutrients, to prevent overloading the blood with too much sugar too soon after eating.

2. Control of the rate of utilization of sugar at the tissue level by the basal metabolic rate, exercise, the climate, the proper amount of insulin receptors on cells and many other cellular mechanisms.

3. The pancreas, located deep in the upper abdomen with both an exocrine (ducts to the outside of the gland) and an endocrine (no ducts-the hormones are taken up directly into the blood capillaries) function, both of which help control blood sugar

4. The permeability of the intestinal tract. This allows nutrients to pass through it and to enter into the cells of the body. These are activities which are controlled carefully. It is surprising to realize that a major function of cells is to block the entry of nutrients not currently needed, and to allow entrance to other nutrients regarded by the cells as necessary at any given moment.

5. The liver is our largest gland. Without it we could only live approximately 12 days. The liver orchestrates all of our chemical processes. It compresses glucose (sugar) into storage blocks called glycogen for efficient and compact longer term storage. Glycogen produced by animals resembles the starch which is produced by plants. Both animal-glycogen and plant-starch are made for carbohydrate storage. As a sugar control mechanism, the liver is not as sensitive as the pancreas, but its function is increased or decreased by blood sugar levels.

6. Temporary storage of sugar. Some foods are processed into sugar by the intestines. This sugar is absorbed from the intestines and then removed from the blood for temporary storage by certain tissues and organs. This sugar is stored until the liver calls for it and compresses it into glycogen. Immediately after a meal the mechanisms involved in this process are working at peak capacity, at a high-powered, rapid pace. This process prevents the blood from becoming syrupy because of the sugar content.

Metabolic disorders involving digestion of food are common in our day. This is because food is so easily obtainable, particularly those concentrated foods that are in a surplus supply. These are generally foods which when overeaten, put a great burden on the metabolic and digestive systems. This burden is felt all the way from the mouth to every digestive organ to completed digestion and the breaking down of nutrients into their simplest forms. There is also a burden placed on the body to eliminate wastes produced from these foods, and to eliminate substances, such as enzymes, which the body manufactures to process the foods. This creates metabolic stress which drains stored energy from the body and is experienced as restlessness, nervousness, fatigue, stiffness, clumsiness and poor concentration. Adaptation to the stress of generating the energy for these tasks puts the body into a state of strain. Finally the body can no longer adapt, and it collapses into the General Adaptation Syndrome (GAS) described by the Canadian physician, Dr. Hans Selye. More recently, this strain and collapse has been referred to as the Accelerated Aging Syndrome, Insulin Resistance or Hyperinsulinism.

The Accelerated Aging Syndrome goes through a course of several steps. The first step is a strain to which the body easily adapts. But continued adaptation results in depletion of reserves. Depletion eventually causes exhaustion. The next step is breakdown, either mental, physical or both. This syndrome is accompanied by accelerated aging and the final event is death.

The operation of this system which deals with the results of overeating causes an effective cellular dehydration and insulin resistance. These subjects are discussed in the following chapters.

*Diabetes And The Hypoglycemic Syndrome - Facts, Findings and Natural Treatments* is about this process. While the words, "accelerated aging" have an ominous ring, the condition is by no means hopeless. If it were, there would be only an academic interest in this subject. But because of our expectation of change, and our belief that a positive course of disease reversal can be immediately set in motion, we have united our efforts in writing this book. It is our wish to acquaint you with the entity of accelerated aging - both the diagnosis of the hypoglycemic syndrome and diabetes - and the methods of treatment, simple practices that can be carried out at home, which offer the only hope for cure.

We pray for God's blessings upon you; that you may become informed about your body and the methods of caring for it. We have made every effort to explain the information in this book clearly enough to enable everyone to understand. Still, there may be some information for which you need further explanation. In this case, your physician or your local library may be able to assist you.

The part of the book most essential for the average reader who is not involved in teaching, is about symptoms and what to do for the disease. Those parts are easily understood, even if you have no interest in the complex biochemistry involved in this very perplexing disorder.

Calvin L. Thrash, Jr., M.D., MPH
Agatha M. Thrash, M.D., FACP

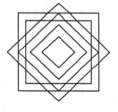

# CHAPTER ONE

# *Diabetes and Hypoglycemia*

### THE EVOLUTION OF THE DISEASE

Disease does not just happen. All disease is due to some kind of transgression of natural law at some time in the history of the person. This transgression, either deliberate or accidental,

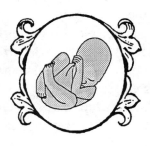

may have occurred several generations back, and may even have been the result of a natural disaster. For example, radiation from the Tunguska Meteorite, eight or nine decades ago, could have caused mutations in genes resulting in a current disability of some kind. This disability could be as minor as a change in an enzyme once capable of digesting dry beans without the production of gas.

Besides radiation, a host of other injurious agents known to damage chromosomes are alcohol, aromatic spices like ginger and pepper, tobacco, coffee and its brown beverage relatives, even if decaffeinated, and many prescription and recreational drugs. Our contemporary lifestyle has drawn a vast amount of attention as a producer of disease. The term "lifestyle" includes diet, good and bad habits, stresses, exercise and recreational choices.

Dr. Hans Selye studied lifestyle diseases for 30 to 40 years, and became the world's leading expert on stress and related diseases. He experimented with many forms of laboratory-induced stress, such as chilling and prolonged fatigue, and found that the body adapts immediately. Substantial changes were noted in blood pressure, blood chemistry and blood flow. He also noted that pupils dilate, muscles develop tension, the mouth goes dry, the strength of the skin changes and many other alterations happen within the body. All of these changes require energy from both the body and the brain.

Adaptation and accommodation to the stresses continues as long as there is stress. But a muscle can hold the tension only as long as it is able to, and then it begins to die. The same thing happens with the chemistry of the blood. We make adaptations as long as we continue to have a storage of energy, but when the stores are depleted, we begin to fail biochemically. Symptoms of chemical failure are nonspecific such as headache, dizziness, fatigue, foggy thinking with a loss of concentration, allergies, emotional upsets, mental symptoms and many more.

The adrenals must also adapt to the stresses by putting out stress hormones. As a result, we can adapt to mild chilling for as long as needed by means of blood vessel changes. This process can require an enormous outlay of chemical energy. Many hormones use cholesterol as a base, such as cortisone and estrogen. Therefore, with any kind of adaptation sufficient to cause stress hormone production, the cholesterol may go up.

Through this mechanism some people acquire a high blood cholesterol, even from a stress as seemingly minor as chilling. The liver must make more cholesterol as raw material for the stress hormones. These changes continue to be made until the stress stops or the adrenals undergo exhaustion. To the pathologist, the size of the adrenals as well as their color announce exhaustion. The normal thickness of the outer layer, called the adrenal cortex, is 1-2mm. In a stressed person it may be 3-4mm. Because the hormones stored in the adrenals have a bright yellow color, the color of the cortex is yellow in a normal person, but will turn tan or brown in a stressed person, after the hormones are used up.

Caffeine use (from drinking coffee, tea or colas and eating chocolate) also causes these adrenal changes. When adrenal exhaustion occurs from repeated and multiplied stresses, the person has a breakdown of some kind. This breakdown can be emotional, social, spiritual, mental or physical. When exhaustion occurs, every experience of life is colored by it. Small irritations suddenly cause pain, whereas before the adaptation exhaustion they were not noticed. Certain smells may now cause nausea, whereas when a person was rested, the same smells were pleasing. Marital discord, trouble on the job, parent-child problems, poor judgment, reduced driving skills and many other distresses or disabilities may surface.

Stress accelerates most disease processes and makes them more difficult and painful. Diseases appear earlier in life when there is prolonged stress. Certainly stress plays a very definite role in illnesses such as diabetes and the hypoglycemic syndrome.

Diabetes, the hypoglycemic syndrome and diseases related to them such as hypertension, cancer, obesity and coronary artery disease, represent the commonest disorders in the United States today. They are true lifestyle disorders and frequently appear together in the same patient. How do they develop? Trace some typical steps many go through, in the following outline:

## *Infancy*
A. Sugar water is administered in the hospital newborn nursery to avoid disturbing sleeping mothers for nursing. This practice introduces newborns to extremely sweet tastes during the first days of life. When a baby is breastfed, the only other liquid that may be needed is plain water, if anything.

B. Early introduction of cow's milk and solid foods anytime during the first three months, will increase the risk of disease.[1] Frequently the foods chosen have free-sugars or fats in them which put a further tax on the infant's immature digestive and immune systems. The great rise in allergies and autoimmune diseases may have their origin in the early introduction of food other than breast milk.

C. A doubling of the birth weight in three to four months instead of the ideal of approximately six months and a tripling in seven to eight months instead of twelve months. Babies are chubby and seem active and happy. This growth acceleration continues at an unnatural pace, mainly due to overfeeding and underexercising, and it leads to the many mental and physical problems listed in the sections below. Somatostatin, a hormone which shuts off the growth hormone, is inhibited by rich food and growth acceleration. Once this process was thought to be desirable, producing attractive, tall men and women. But it is now known that this process leads to early maturity, school dropouts, premature aging and a host of lifestyle disorders.

## *Childhood*

A. Mentally, growth accelerated children are usually very bright, ahead of their years.

B. Physically, these children are large, well rounded and husky, yet they sometimes complain of fatigue. They often don't enjoy physical activities such as running or other very active sports. Physical challenges may or may not interest or inspire them. Some will push themselves to excel in sports.

C. They may often feel that they "cannot wait" for meals.

D. They generally eat heartily at meals and also frequently between meals.

E. They usually love sweets and all other rich foods.

F. Socially they are often leaders in everything, involved in many kinds of activities and excel in their studies.

## *Adolescence*

A. The accelerated physical and mental progression continues on through childhood. Huskiness may then turn into fat and some adolescents go through a period struggling with overweight.

B. While young men may be affected as well as young women, the syndrome is more likely to be recognized earlier in young women because of the nature of a woman's physiological changes and stresses. This syndrome does not generally appear in men until they have reached their late thirties or forties.

C. Young women may find at this time, that they suddenly recognize an emotionally blue period which only lasts a few hours and occurs infrequently at first. Menstrual periods usually begin at any time from nine to twelve years.

These young women are often good students early in life and are generally tall, attractive and popular. Because of the early maturation of the body before developing experience with life, a certain percentage of them will develop a rebellious spirit, become uncontrollable or wild and most likely will drop out of school. Some may join one of many counter-culture movements.

## *Young Adult*

A. Many of these young women marry well and immediately have a period of disabling fatigue which results in depression. When the first baby arrives, they find themselves more energy-drained than they had expected. The attention needed for the baby tends to make them disregard their discomfort. Another baby may be expected before the mothers are ready for a second child. These women may now have reached a point where they are experiencing a change in their disposition. The first serious depression may appear, a frightening state of mind over which they have no control and which they can no longer easily dismiss. Appetite usually remains good and they have moments when they are especially energetic and will tend to compulsively overwork.

B. Single men and women follow the same general pattern. They have great plans and expectations and every hope and belief in their ability to accomplish them. But their dreams remain fruitless because their mental and physical energies begin to deteriorate for reasons they cannot explain. On days when they seem to have more energy, they will drive themselves to accomplish their tasks.

## Beginning to Fail

A. Husbands begin to complain that the house is not cared for, even though they know their wives like a neat home. The women may not have the energy to maintain a system of orderly housekeeping, and the home is usually cluttered and disorganized.

B. The wives are frequently out-of-sorts. They are disappointed to discover they are not the superwomen they thought themselves to be.

C. Hypoglycemic wives generally need much encouragement and reassurance from their husbands. But their husbands may be afraid to give them encouragement because they fear they will make them too dependent.

D. The women tend to develop exacting personalities and will have many emotional and physical problems.

## Signs of Failure

A. At about the same time the signs of physical or emotional breakdown are seen in women, approximately in their late thirties and forties, the syndrome begins to rapidly develop in men. The twenty years in which women have been gradually showing more and more signs of illness are condensed into two or three years for men. Both men and women begin to gain weight and have no energy to keep up social or business engagements. They start to withdraw from most of the activities they once found gratifying.

B. The wife's housework or the husband's occupation suffer from lack of organization. Neither seems able to finish any projects they have begun, and unfinished work begins to accumulate.

C. The suffering person finally tells the spouse there is something seriously wrong. A woman may consider suicide, divorce or running away from home. A man may consider changing his profession, moving to another city, divorce, suicide or running away. A new mate is sometimes seen as a solution to problems which appear to have no other solution. But the new mate is found to have the same, or perhaps different, "intolerable flaws."

## Mental Signs

A. Depression. The doctor feels a woman's ovaries are depleted and prescribes estrogen, a tranquilizer or both.

B. Lack of concentration. Previously bright children or adolescents become poor students or poor employees. Employees may be labeled "burnouts."

C. Men who have been attentive and orderly in their business and social responsibilities, begin to forget things and are told they need a vacation or a tranquilizer.

D. Women cannot organize themselves or their activities long enough to plan and execute housework. They become so easily distracted that any interruption, even a phone call, turns into a time-consuming diversion. Physicians often believe these women need to see a psychiatrist. They may also make recommendations for surgery on their female organs. Many physicians mistakenly believe that these measures will clear up the women's problems.

## *Wide Mood Swings*

A. Many sufferers have wide mood swings, often from one extreme to another, in the same hour.

B. Occasionally a person will have bizarre thoughts. One patient was plagued with fears and imagined putting her child into the washing machine. She appeared to have serious doubts about her sanity, but because she believed she was not mentally ill, she trusted she would not act on her imaginings. Her husband also questioned her sanity, but he had no reassurance that she would not behave in a bizarre manner. A psychiatrist accepted her as a patient and wanted to treat her with tranquilizers, shock treatments or a hospitalization.

C. Compulsions develop.
    1. To talk about the illness.
    2. To talk of doctors and pill schedules.
    3. Repetitious activities sometimes begin, such as handwashing, daily shopping trips and overspending, interminable vacuuming, many telephone calls, constant visiting and coffee drinking, furniture moving, paper shuffling but no purposeful desk work, etc..

There are many variations in the development of this serious metabolic process. Perhaps your story was not included or described exactly here. But you may find other diagnostic clues in one of the following chapters. The next several chapters will discuss diabetes with a section on the hypoglycemic syndrome following.

While we do not like to hear the term "accelerated aging," it is clear that this is the pattern of events and "accelerated aging" is the result. Infants and children are force-fed by well-meaning adults until they develop metabolic and structural changes. These changes cause the entire life experience to be compressed into fewer years than the natural growth process should have and produces havoc in the process.

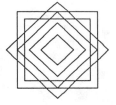

# CHAPTER TWO

# Diabetes Defined

It is important to recognize that there are two major types of diabetes. They are similar, and yet in many ways so different they seem to be two different diseases. They were formerly known as juvenile onset and adult onset diabetes. More recent usage and the preferred terminology is Type I or insulin-dependent diabetes mellitus (IDDM or juvenile), and Type II or non-insulin-dependent diabetes mellitus (NIDDM or adult). As the names suggest, the Type I diabetic has an absolute deficiency of insulin and always requires insulin injections as a part of his or her treatment regimen; whereas the Type II patient may have an abundance of insulin and may never actually require insulin in order to live. The Type II disease should be controllable by careful regulation of diet and lifestyle-related factors.

This does not mean to imply that the lifestyle of the Type I patient is unimportant - far from it, as conscientious control of diet, exercise, weight and regularity in all activities of life will add years to the life of the insulin-dependent diabetic. These factors will also preserve, for a much longer period, the faculties of vision, hearing, balance, coordination, sensation in the extremities and the quality of life. Type I diabetes is more difficult to manage because it requires professional help. Type II diabetes can usually be managed at home by the patient, using home remedies.

Fortunately, Type I diabetes is much less common than Type II. In Type I, complications tend to be more severe and occur at younger ages than in Type II. Just a few years ago, the average juvenile diabetic could not expect to live many years past the twenties, with severe complications making the last years miserable. Now, with increased knowledge of the rational use of insulin coupled with a knowledge of the necessary lifestyle changes, a Type I diabetic can often look forward to a nearly normal lifespan.

## Complications

It is the complications of both of these types of diabetes that make them such dreaded illnesses for both the patient and the physician. Complications include diabetic ketoacidosis (severe chemical derangement with acid in the blood, due to uncontrolled diabetes and the body's attempts at adjustment), which can be followed by diabetic coma if it is not corrected immediately. Coma is a medical emergency that will result in death in a few days unless treated rapidly and vigorously.

Ketosis (a reaction very similar to starvation caused by using body fat) is not particularly harmful if it is arrested before it develops into ketoacidosis. For a Type I diabetic, insulin must be administered. In the Type II diabetic this ketosis may also be brought on by fasting and can be ended by eating.

Diabetic ketoacidosis may result from unusual and/or prolonged stress to the body such as that caused by illness, an accident, surgery or emotional stress. The immediate effects of stress and the beginning of the progression of ketoacidosis begins with elevated blood sugar followed by sugar in the urine. Stress hormones increase the blood sugar level by lowering the insulin supply. When the insulin supply is decreased and no longer available, sugar cannot be used as a source of energy, so that fats must be used instead. By-products of fat metabolism, the ketones, back up into the blood. They acidify the blood which leads to ketoacidosis.[2]

Large amounts of water are put out with the sugar and volumes of urine are passed. The person develops an unquenchable thirst and chronic dehydration. Yeast vaginitis may develop with itching. Because of the rich sugar level in the skin and blood, other infections may occur such as pyelonephritis (kidney infection), bladder and skin infections, mouth and eye infections, etc.. Increased fat breakdown causes ketones and other by-products of fat breakdown, called acetones, to bring on symptoms of nausea or loss of appetite. The symptoms progress to drowsiness, then coma. As this occurs, a fruity odor on the breath of the diabetic, caused by the acetones, can be noticed by other people.

These complications are typically problems of the Type I diabetic. The Type II diabetic will usually develop ketoacidosis only with the most severe diseases such as life-threatening infections. Most Type II diabetics are quite stable biochemically, even when the blood sugar is quite high.

Insulin shock, from too much insulin, from too much or unexpected exercise, or not enough food, is always a dreaded possibility in the insulin-user and it may be life-threatening. Even the milder instances of insulin reactions may cause subtle but permanent damage to the brain and nervous system, as well as causing accidents due to mental lapses. It is critically important not to take too much insulin.

A study recently reported (June 1993, not yet published) indicates that the "tighter" the control of blood sugar with insulin, the less complications of diabetes.

Other complications common to both types are largely related to problems of the blood vessels, circulation, and the nervous system. In the eyes, damaged capillaries and arterioles cause hemorrhages in the retina and other areas of the eyes, often leading to impaired sight or blindness. The optic nerve and its fibers can degenerate and cataracts may occur prematurely, usually requiring surgery, sometimes at quite an early age.

Glaucoma may sometimes complicate diabetes. This condition consists of increased pressure in the eyes which can lead to visual symptoms and eventually blindness. It tends to run in families and is the cause of blindness in one-tenth of all cases of blindness in the United States. High blood pressure, overweight, diabetes, use of corticosteroid medications and other factors can all lead to glaucoma. The treatment is given in our books on home remedies (See Bibliography.), and starts with the same treatment given for high blood pressure. As the blood pressure goes up, the likelihood of glaucoma also goes up. (See Chapter Ten for instructions on reducing the blood pressure.)

Damaged coronary vessels predispose a diabetic to increased risk of heart attacks, while diseased vessels feeding the brain lead to an increased risk of strokes. Circulatory problems in the extremities are well-known, often causing infection, gangrene, and loss of feet or legs. Injuries to the glomeruli, the tiny filtration apparatus of the kidney that purifies the blood, and to capillaries can lead to kidney failure, with no recourse other than renal dialysis and the hope that a kidney transplant may be possible.

The following chart lists symptoms of which you should be aware and take actions to treat.

### Signs of Type I Complications
### When Diabetes Is Uncontrolled

Acute Signs
- Acetone - fruity breath odor
- Infections of all kinds
- Insulin shock or low blood sugar
- Ketoacidosis
- Large volumes of water drunk
- Large volumes of urine produced
- Weight loss but large appetite
- Loss of appetite

Longterm Complications
- Cataracts
- Early blood vessel deterioration
- Early nerve and brain deterioration
- Gangrene in feet
- Heart attacks
- Kidney failure
- Osteoporosis
- Strokes

## Diabetic Gangrene

One of the most troublesome complications of diabetes relates to reduced blood flow to the feet and legs. (See Chapter Six for "Daily Care of the Feet.")

## Case History

Victor Andrews, age 49 and suffering with hypertension, came to Uchee Pines Lifestyle Center with a three year history of diabetes. He was taking 40 units of insulin daily plus a diuretic for hypertension. Because of pain when he walked, his surgeon had done a bypass operation on the aorta near the terminal branch, into the two leg arteries. The surgery was successful for only three months. Now, he had the beginnings of gangrene in both feet. His left foot had a two inch zone of purple discoloration just under his ankle bone, with a one inch ulceration in the center. The second toe was dark purple and the side of his foot had a 2 inch blister filled with bloody fluid.

The blister ruptured the day he arrived. Finger pressure anywhere on the skin of his foot required 31 seconds for the blood to run back into the fingerprint. His former doctor had told him to go home and take pain pills until the gangrene had fully developed. The gangrene was expected to progress with so much pain and discomfort, that Victor would become willing to have his leg amputated. It was at this time that Victor heard of us and came to see if we could help him save his leg. His right foot, which was in better condition than his left foot, had only a single wet ulcer on the great toe.

We began his treatment program immediately: exercise, a salt-free, total vegetarian diet, warm charcoal foot baths for 20 minutes twice a day, charcoal by mouth for high blood cholesterol, massage to his arms, trunk, thighs and upper legs and herbal remedies. The herbal remedies we used included two or three cloves of garlic with each meal, for its antibacterial effects and its anticlotting properties, to protect his feet from blood clots. He drank White Willow Bark tea for his pain and Hawthorn Berry tea for his hypertension. Because of the positive effects of the diet and the teas, he was able to stop taking his blood pressure medicine. We gave him Dandelion tea as an herbal diuretic.

Normally, Victor drank wine or beer several times a week and smoked a pack of cigarettes daily. He was willing to stop the alcohol and asked for help to quit his smoking habit. We explained to him how both of these unhealthful habits damage the interior of blood vessels and promote circulatory problems. With a great deal of effort, he was able to stop these two habits.

He could only walk ten steps before getting pain in his calves and feet. He would then be forced to sit down and rest. He started a program of walking in open-toe shoes, selected calisthenics and other out-door exercises, plus hoeing and transplanting in the garden, digging post holes and using a pruning saw. Being outdoors was also a part of his treatment. He made cuts in a pair of shoes to relieve pressure on the gangrenous portions of his feet.

At first he did not enjoy the vegetarian food and liked being salt-free even less. But he felt triumphant when the blood pressure pills could be stopped. By the seventh day he was tolerating the food better and even beginning to say he liked certain dishes. Breakfast consisted of fruits and whole grains, and lunch was made up of vegetables and whole grains. Both meals contained two tablespoons of seeds or nuts, prepared in a variety of sauces, spreads, gravies, milks or toppings. His supper consisted only of Echinacea tea to strengthen his immune system. A two-meal plan is much preferred over a three-meal plan. The two-meal plan promotes weight loss, good digestion and sweet, restful sleep. It also increases the strength of the immune system.

Victor was given one tablespoon of charcoal internally four times a day to lower cholesterol and adsorb toxins from tissue deterioration in his feet. Charcoal adsorbs toxins and infectious agents and may carry some oxygen to the tissues when applied externally. Evidence exists that charcoal may also help lower blood sugar.

First thing every morning we prepared a charcoal foot bath in which he soaked his feet for 30-60 minutes. Because of the severity of the arterial disease in his legs, we did not make his charcoal foot baths warmer than 100-101 degrees. Hot water can cause the tissue metabolism to rise, resulting in the need for more oxygen, but the arteries cannot deliver additional blood to supply this need. Due to the infection in the sores, we wanted to try to get some warming of the skin, at least up to body temperature, as the best healing occurs at body temperature. His feet were constantly cold because of poor circulation. We made warm herbal foot baths using Goldenseal and Garlic teas to heal the ulcers. These were given at mid-day.

We prepared a third foot bath with Comfrey once a day. He received a light fingertip massage to the healthiest areas of his feet after each bath, to promote circulation. The Comfrey wash provided an active ingredient, allantoin, which encourages healing.

At midday we applied hot compresses to his groin area to encourage blood flow to his feet. Applying a compress to one part of the body to increase blood flow, in hopes that this measure will reflexively help another part is a common technique. Every evening at bedtime Victor got a backrub and leg and arm massage for circulation and sleep.

We gave him blueberry tea for his diabetes, Ginkgo tea for circulation, and three antibiotic herbs: two to three cloves of Garlic with each meal and one cup of Goldenseal and one cup of Chaparral tea per day.

In three weeks he could walk two miles a day, the first quarter mile without pain, and there were obvious signs of healing in both feet. His blood pressure was down to normal and his blood sugar readings were greatly improved, even though we had cut back his insulin dosage to five units twice per day. In two months his finger-pressure-pallor on the big toe was only two seconds! We were pleased. His insulin dose was down from 40 units to only 10.

Eventually, all of his skin lesions healed, he returned to his home in a northern state and did well on the program for four years. Then suddenly he became depressed. He indulged himself by eating sugary junk foods and returned to smoking and drinking beer. After six months he had to have his left foot and leg amputated, and five months later his right foot and leg were amputated. Two weeks after the last amputation, he had a heart attack from which he never recovered. Within three months his brother-in-law called to tell us of his death.

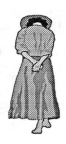

## *Diabetic Neuropathy*

In diabetes, all areas of the nervous system may be affected, including the brain, the motor and sensory nerves and the autonomic nervous system. Symptoms range from mild to very severe pain, burning and tingling. Often there can be nearly complete loss of sensation in the feet, causing small injuries to go unnoticed, leading to infection and gangrene. Involvement of nerves to the gastrointestinal tract and the heart can cause strange symptoms such as sudden sharp pains, diarrhea at night, constipation alternating with diarrhea and other problems.

Bladder and/or anal sphincter control may be lost. Impotence is common in men. Loss of sympathetic nervous system tone can make it difficult to control the blood pressure, causing fainting when the patient stands up. Brain involvement can mimic mental disorders and serious neurological disease. Strangely, the nerve symptoms can occur as one of the first signals of diabetes, at times when the blood sugar is only slightly elevated.

In standard medicine prior to 1990, there was virtually no hope for improvement in diabetic neuropathy. But we discovered many years ago in our Lifestyle Center, that modifying lifestyle factors results in slow, but often striking improvements in these formerly untreatable disorders. The mainstays of treatment involve the use of a totally vegetarian diet (no milk, eggs, cheese or meat), high in fiber and low in fat, emphasizing foods high in myo-inositol, a vitamin-like substance wasted by diabetics through their kidneys and found in plentiful supply in certain foods (See Chapter Ten for a list of foods high in myo-inositol.), exercise to tolerance and strict regularity in all things.

### Case History of Diabetic Neuropathy and Erythrocytosis

Inez Stewart, a dear lady in her late 50's, came to Uchee Pines complaining bitterly of shooting pains in her thighs and severe burning in her whole body. She was so miserable and anxious, she had not been able to smile for over a year. During the past year, she had been hospitalized twice, with four other visits to the emergency room for treatment of intolerable pain. Except for the times when powerful painkillers or narcotics were given to her, she had no relief from the overwhelming pain.

Her doctor had studied her condition using a complete blood count and blood sugar tests. He did not recognize her blood sugar problem because her fasting blood sugar was only 114. Her hemoglobin was 14.4 grams. He decided she was healthy and only had a problem with menopausal hysteria. He prescribed estrogen. She felt worse taking the hormones and stopped them after two months. A variety of drugs were then prescribed for her, none of which alleviated her symptoms.

When she arrived at our Lifestyle Center, we thoroughly evaluated her case. The first diagnosis we made was erythrocytosis (the opposite of anemia). The first treatment we prescribed, even before her blood sugar levels had been thoroughly tested, was to have her donate a pint of blood to the Red Cross. This brought her hemoglobin down below 14 grams and allowed her blood to circulate more freely. When the blood is too rich and heavy, the circulation is slowed down. Women living at an elevation of 5000 feet or below should have an ideal hemoglobin level between 10.5 and 12.5. After that the higher the hemoglobin level, the more likely a woman will suffer from fatigue.

Two hours after breakfast we took a blood sample from her for a sugar level. Her sugar level was 132. We consider any reading over 100 at two hours after eating to be suggestive of diabetes, so we made a diagnosis of diabetes. Her pains and misery were all caused by diabetic neuropathy complicated by stress erythrocytosis. Stress erythrocytosis is a condition caused by the presence of too many red blood cells. This overproduction is generated by the stresses of disease, lifestyle or emotions and results in a slowed down circulation.

Inez was so sick and disorganized in her thinking, she could not even get a glass of water for herself. Sitting through church, or even a 20 minute lecture, was out of the question for her. She tried to make it through the night without calling for help, but most mornings she could not stand the pain and anxiety past 4:30 or 5:00. "Isn't there something you can do for me?" she would ask us. "I can't stand it another minute!" We would give her sedative and pain-relieving teas (See Chapter Twelve.), and put her in a cool, sedative bath at 97-98 degrees.

The diet we prepared for her concentrated on foods high in myo-inositol (See Chapter Eleven). By the fifth week she was improved enough to call her husband and ask him to drive the 350 miles for a visit. She met him in the front yard with a smile. He took her by the hand and began looking for me immediately. When he found me, he walked into the room with a big smile and said, "This is the first smile I have seen on my wife's face in over a year."

By the eighth week she was walking 8 miles a day and had lost about 12 pounds, which brought her to a normal weight. Her neuropathy was 60-70% better and she thought she could start helping with the work at the Institute. She stayed about six months and during this entire period she was extremely careful with her diet. When a dish was passed around the table, no matter how appetizing it appeared or how hungry she was, she would not eat it if she were not 100% certain it fit into her diet.

This case illustrates several good points. The first point is that people who have suffered severely, who gain improvements from diet and exercise, will not complain if they cannot have this or that food or do this or that activity. They are so thankful to be better they almost never grieve over their restrictions.

Secondly, mild diabetics can have severe neuropathy. The third point is that stress erythrocytosis often complicates chronic disease. Chronic dehydration and concentration of blood occurs with diabetes. (See discussion of Chronic Dehydration in Chapter Ten.) And the fourth point is diabetic neuropathy can be cured using natural and physiologic remedies, whereas standard medicine as yet has no specific treatment.

## Foot Ulcers

Another complication often found in diabetes is chronic foot ulcers. These often refuse to heal. They can extend into muscle and connective tissue planes and eventually cause osteomyelitis, an infection of the bone, which may make it necessary for surgery.

## Case History

A 45 year-old West Indian man who had been insulin dependent for the past eight years, came to our Lifestyle Center with a large, painful, chronic, open ulcer on his left big toe. This ulcer had eaten away at the bone and had a foul odor. It extended by a large, closed channel which burrowed about five inches under his skin, from the big toe, to the beginning of the heel pad, involving much of the sole of his foot. His physician in the West Indies had recommended amputation but our patient was hoping his foot would heal with carefully applied hydrotherapy. We had very little hope, but immediately began warm water foot soaks at 102 degrees in charcoal water, alternating every five minutes with cold water at 70 degrees for 30 seconds. These soaks yielded no recognizable benefit other than deodorizing.

Our staff physicians evaluated his foot and reached the unanimous opinion that he would require a below-the-knee amputation. We felt that nothing less extensive would ever heal. He refused to consider an amputation, saying he believed the Lord would save his foot, even though he felt he might lose his big toe.

To help him accept our opinion, we sent him to an orthopedist who thoroughly tested his blood vessel capabilities. This doctor told the patient he could decide right then for a below-the-knee amputation or wait for the "rotten foot" to completely poison his system. This meant he could take a chance on living another month or six weeks with it until it killed him with toxicity and infection.

The patient still refused the surgery. He believed the Lord would heal him. We all prayed for his life and asked the Lord to give us wisdom to manage such a serious case. He developed a fever and anemia (his hemoglobin was 7.9, which is a little over half the usual 12.75 - 14.5 ideal for men). We redoubled our efforts. He could not walk, so his exercise consisted of arm exercises and straight leg-raises. We began to pack the ulcer and the channel underneath with sugar wet down with povidone-iodine, a common microbicide from the drug store, used for antiseptic purposes on the skin. Pure sugar inhibits bacterial growth, a quality known and used for preserving fruit. It is not absorbed through the skin to affect the blood sugar. Twice a day the ulcer and channel were irrigated and packed. We continued the hot and cold water soaks just before each irrigation. To reduce systemic toxicity, he received a heaping tablespoon of charcoal by mouth every four hours.

After the first week he appeared to be no worse, so we began to believe we might be staying ahead of the blood poisoning and infection, but we still had no hope for healing. After two weeks, the patient reported reduction of pain and a lessening of the swelling. His wife confirmed her faith in these signs as the beginning of his healing. One month later, physical evidences of healing could be seen. He eventually lost his big toe, but his foot healed, and his leg was saved. We felt divine power had combined with human effort, to save the leg of this man of great faith.

## Blindness

Visual difficulties, which affect 50% of diabetics within 10 years of diagnosis and 80% within 15 years, are another serious complication of diabetes. Microaneurysms, which are tiny balloonlike swellings on capillaries, and hemorrhages occur in the retina and encourage retinal separation. Hypertension and stress erythrocytosis (See Index.) make it worse. Often laser surgery is used in an attempt to save the retina. The retina will sometimes function well after surgery. But sometimes the retinal disease progresses to the point of blindness. Smoking, coffee, tea, colas, alcohol and uncontrolled diabetes all accelerate progression of this disorder.

## Other Complications

Urinary tract infections, kidney disease, sometimes progressing to kidney failure, mouth and skin problems such as fungus infections and irritations of the genital area, rashes and pyorrhea are sometimes complications of diabetes.

Airline pilots must control diabetes by diet alone or be grounded. Diabetes ranks third as a cause of medical grounding. If a pilot requires insulin, then his diabetes is considered serious enough to result in such problems as hypoglycemia, causing reduced mental functioning and poor judgment.

### Case History

A 51 year-old pilot with a fasting blood sugar level of 310 mg% went on a spare diet of 160gm. carbohydrates, 90gm. protein and 60gm. of fats. He took only two meals daily and had nothing to eat after 3:00 pm. The emphasis was on green vegetables and fruits. He avoided desserts, empty calorie foods and caloric drinks such as fruit juices and sodas. His health improved rapidly and within 8 weeks he had brought his fasting blood sugar level down to 130. In 16 weeks, the level was consistently below 100.

This case illustrates the fact that a spare diet can be successful. Animal protein has a diabetogenic and an atherogenic effect (promotes hardening of the arteries), and will promote acceleration of aging. We always prescribe a vegan vegetarian diet which includes total avoidance of meat, milk, eggs and cheese.

## Diabetes Management

People with diabetes are twice as likely to have heart disease and to develop it earlier in life, than those without diabetes. The increased risk is due to the greater predisposition diabetics have for atherosclerosis, hypertension and high cholesterol. Diabetes management, therefore, must include reduction of all controllable risks as follows:

1. Reduce low-density lipoprotein cholesterol (LDL) in the blood with a diet that has no animal products of any kind. Free fats (mayonnaise, oils, margarine, nut and seed butters) must also be avoided unless underweight is a problem. You may use up to two tablespoons of nuts or seeds with each meal. Commercial mayonnaise should never be used. (See our cookbook, *Eat For Strength*, for recipes for no-fat spreads.)

   LDL promotes accumulation of fats in the arteries, while HDL removes fats from blood and tissues. High density lipoprotein cholesterol (HDL), the "good cholesterol," can be increased with exercise, weight reduction and stopping smoking. Exercise should begin with walking and progress as quickly as the patient can tolerate, until an hour a day is spent in vigorous (but not violent) exercise.

2. Control stress through religious experience, exercise and reduction of stressors. (See Chapter 10 for Stress Control Measures)

3. Control hypertension by appropriate diet, exercise and herbal teas. (See Chapter Ten for the section, "How to Bring the Blood Pressure Down." Also see "Hypertension" in our books, *Home Remedies* and *Natural Treatments for High Blood Pressure*.)

4. Stop the smoking habit. Smoking intensifies all risks in diabetes and must not be a part of the diabetic's lifestyle.

5. Overweight is an enemy and should be avoided. (see Chapter Ten for weight-control method)

## Diagnostic Criteria

Since 1980, specialists in diabetes in the United States have made far-reaching changes in the interpretation of diagnostic criteria for diabetes. The changes have involved rather drastic revisions in the blood sugar level at which physicians diagnose diabetes. We believe these changes in criteria have caused a delay in treatment for those who need early lifestyle changes to avoid developing a serious case of diabetes. The term "carbohydrate intolerance" has been coined and the blood sugar level at which diabetes is diagnosed has been raised, leaving true diabetics who have lower blood sugar levels, undiagnosed.

We feel this trend was dictated by the fact that virtually the entire nation has undergone an increase in blood sugar levels, perhaps due to overeating and deteriorating lifestyles. We find this diagnostic trend regrettable. One authority, when the new criteria were announced, made the ironic remark, "Now our patients will be dying of carbohydrate intolerance instead of diabetes!"

A remarkable article was printed in the January 1988 issue of the **Southern Medical Journal** entitled "Diabetic Glomerulosclerosis Without Concurrent Diabetes Mellitus," in which the patient was clearly a diabetic by the older criteria. Use of the liberal criteria will lead to other strange and confusing articles in medical journals, as well as depriving physicians and health educators of the early warning signs essential for early diagnosis and prevention. The diagnostic criteria referred to later in this booklet are the older, tried-and-true ones that have served the medical community well for many years. With these reliable criteria, we try to predict a tendency toward diabetes 20 years before a person breaks down with a crippling disease and try to reverse this tendency before any damage is done.

People who are beginning to show signs of accelerated aging, such as elevated cholesterol, a fasting blood sugar over 90 or 95, reduced immune resistance, repeated kidney infections, mouth infections or wide mood swings, should be suspected of early or pre-diabetes. A person labeled with this term needs to take the matter just as seriously as if labeled with diabetes, (which in fact, it is) and give it careful thought and attention.

## The Glucose Tolerance Test

### One Method of Diagnosis of Diabetes

The patient arrives at the laboratory after fasting for at least 6 hours. Samples of blood are tested while the patient is still fasting, then 30 minutes after taking a loading dose of glucose (200 gm), one hour later, and at two, three, four, and five hours.

The highest reading of the blood sugar after a meal should be no higher than 70 mg. above the fasting level. The difference between the highest and lowest values after meals should be no less than 50 nor greater than 80 mg%. If it is higher or lower, we should make the diagnosis of probable hypoglycemia or diabetes. The extent to which this difference is exceeded either way represents the severity of the metabolic disorder. Even when symptoms (food-relieved weakness, junk food responsive symptoms) are not substantiated by blood tests, hypoglycemia cannot be ruled out.

### Second Method of Diagnosis in Diabetes

Diabetes is definite if fasting blood sugar is over 120 on two readings, the one hour after-meal reading is over 170, or the two hour reading after-meal is over 130. At the lower readings the case is mild; at the higher readings the case is more severe.

### Third Method of Diagnosis in Diabetes

Add the laboratory readings for these four tests (fasting, 30 minute, one and two-hour-after-meal specimens). If the GTS (glucose tolerance sum) is less than 500, diabetes is not present, 800 and over means diabetes. Between 650 and 800, there is a 95% probability. Between 500 and 650 is borderline.

## Indications For Doing A Glucose Tolerance Test

Since we perform glucose tolerance tests very rarely now, we have set certain guidelines which help us decide which cases may need this expensive, and sometimes physically taxing test.

1. When the history is typical for diabetes or hypoglycemic syndrome, but the fasting and 2-hour post-prandial (after-meal) blood sugar levels are inconclusive.

2. Even when history is not typical, if the fasting blood sugar is over 100, and the 2-hour blood sugar levels are inconclusive. If the fasting blood sugar is over 95, there is a 50% chance of an abnormality in the glucose tolerance test. Over 100 there is a 75% chance, and over 105 it is almost certain that the glucose tolerance test will have at least some degree of abnormality.

## Preparation For The Glucose Tolerance Test

1. Avoid low calorie or weight reducing diets for at least three days before the test, as these may cause the body to overreact.

### Normal Glucose Tolerance Curve

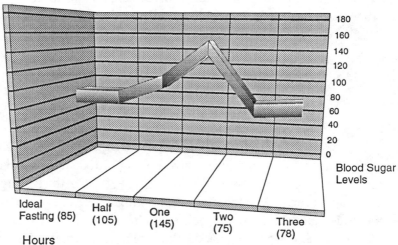

| | 180 |
| 160 |
| 140 |
| 120 |
| 100 |
| 80 |
| 60 |
| 40 |
| 20 |
| 0 |

Blood Sugar Levels

Ideal Fasting (85)  Half (105)  One (145)  Two (75)  Three (78)

Hours

2. Carefully follow a high carbohydrate diet, including plenty of potatoes, fruits, vegetables and whole grain breads and cereals for three days prior to the test.

3. Avoid alcohol for three days before the test.

4. During the fast and during the test there should be no smoking, no drinking of coffee or other brown beverages and no use of any other drugs.

5. Postpone the test if an acute illness occurs.

6. Do no vigorous exercise immediately before or during the test. Similarly, avoid bed rest during the test, if possible.

7. Fast the entire night before the test and continue the fast until after the test is completed.

8. Response to the glucose load given in the laboratory is different for mornings and afternoons. The test must be performed in the morning, because the readings will change in the afternoons, and the diagnostic criteria are based on morning readings.

## *Preparation For The Two-Hour Post-Prandial Test*

1. Follow instructions one through six for Glucose Tolerance Test above.

2. On the test day, eat a large breakfast. Two hours 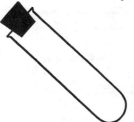 later, blood will be drawn. If the plasma glucose level is above 150, the diagnosis is diabetes. If it is between 90 and 150, it is suspect.

   We expect the blood sugar level to be below the fasting level at two hours.

## *Results of Increased Blood Sugar*

It is not a minor matter to have fasting blood sugar levels high; even to a small degree above ideals of 70-85 in the fasting state, and over 150 at one hour after eating. Here are some of the consequences of high blood sugar.

1. Increased adhesiveness of blood platelets causing a greater likelihood of blood-clotting inside veins.

2. Increase in uric acid blood levels promoting gout, a form of arthritis
3. Increase in blood triglycerides, a type of blood fat.
4. Increase in blood cholesterol, another blood fat.
5. Increase in free fatty acids in atheromatous plaques which build up in arteries causing heart and artery disease.
6. Increase in blood cortisol levels. (Blood cortisol is a hormone produced in the adrenals in response to stress.)
7. Increase in body weight.
8. Reduction in phagocytic index; the ability of the white blood cells to eat germs.
9. Reduction in the number of insulin receptors on cells, which promotes production of high insulin levels in the blood. The high insulin causes the release of nor-epinephrine which can cause hypertension.

## Causes of Urine Sugar Reading Errors

The use of the following substances can alter the chemical reactivity of urine glucose, resulting in underestimation of urine glucose levels. These chemicals can put substances in the urine that inhibit the indicator used to determine urine sugar.

Ampicillin
Ascorbic Acid
Aspirin
Bisacodyl (Dulcolax)
Caffeine (coffee, colas, tea and chocolate)
Chloral Hydrate
Darvon Compound

Diazepam (Valium)

Digoxin (Lanoxin)
Ferrous Sulphate
Flurazepam (Dalmane)
Furosemide (Lasix)
Phenacetin
Phenobarbital
Prednisone
Propoxyphene Hydrochloride
Secobarbital (Seconal)

## Incidence

There is little doubt that both heredity and environment play quite significant roles in both Type I and Type II diabetes. The exact roles of each have not been completely defined, but knowledge is increasing. In the case of Type II diabetics, it is becoming clear that even a strong genetic predisposition will not usually bring on the disease unless there are damaging lifestyle factors.

Likewise, in Type I, it appears that only certain people who have had an infection with a virus such as Coxsackie B, rubella, mumps, etc., will have their pancreatic beta cells affected and only if they have the genetic predisposition. It seems that an autoimmune chain reaction sets up to cause destruction of the beta cells and the onset of Type I diabetes. This has led to the bizarre specter of the conventional attempt to use cortisone-type drugs and immunosuppressants to try to stop the process. There has to be a better way, one which will not endanger the life and health of a person by the use of hazardous drugs.

## Insulin Dependent Diabetes Mellitus (IDDM) - Type I

Type I diabetes was formerly called juvenile diabetes. A recent study highlighted the fact that not much is known about predisposing factors. From 1978-1980 an international study group gathered information from diabetic registries in 18 countries with a total of 31 centers. They found that the incidence varied markedly within the 18 nations.

The main variable proved to be climatic; i.e., the colder the weather, the more diabetes. The incidence varied from 0.6/100,000 in Japan to 29.5/100,000 in Finland. In the U.S. the incidence ranged from 9.4 in San Diego to 20.8 in Rochester, Minnesota. In the U.S., 22,000 children developed IDDM during the study period. If the incidence were the same in the U.S. as in Japan, only 2,700 children would have the disease. Two large studies in Sweden and Finland are currently investigating the role of viral and dietary determinants in colder climates. "Not much attention is being given to lifestyle factors so far."[3]

Lifestyle factors include clothing. Chilling of the body, an often overlooked event, is a stress which begins in infancy and happens more often with more detrimental effects in colder climates. Mothers need instruction on the proper clothing of infants and youth. The entire body of a child should be warmly clothed, with special care taken to keep the limbs and shoulders warmly covered. Tight bands around the waist should always be avoided, as this cuts off circulation, hinders breathing and puts unnecessary pressure on internal organs.

An interesting study from Finland showed that the higher the coffee consumption, the higher the incidence of IDDM. The colder countries of Scandinavia have the highest coffee consumption in the world.[4]

Some researchers have called attention to the fact that where the use of dairy products is high, IDDM is also high. Some precipitating factor may be present in dairy milk which triggers the genetic weakness to degenerate the pancreatic islet cells. Cow's milk fed to infants before the age of six months increases the likelihood of later development of diabetes.

At the time the climate studies were done, nothing was known about the possible relationship of milk and diabetes. Milk consumption in the colder countries tends to be higher than in the more tropical climates. More investigation is needed about the relationship of climate, milk consumption and diabetes.

Dr. Carolyn Berdanier described the interaction of genetics and nutrition in determining the incidence of obesity and diabetes.[5] In her experiments on rats she showed the expression of diabetes to be dependent on the type of diet such animals were fed. In fact, her data clearly showed diet to have a major role in determining if the diabetes would be expressed in these genetically predisposed animals.

Martin and coworkers produced studies showing dietary protein as a possible "trigger." They found milk, and particularly skim milk to be diabetogenic, even when present in only 1% of the diet (that would be about as much as the salt added to the average diet). They found also that wheat gluten is capable of initiating the insulin-dependent syndrome.[6]

## Non-Insulin Dependent Diabetes Mellitus (NIDDM) - Type II

NIDDM has been ascribed to a number of lifestyle-related factors: obesity, inactivity, diets rich in fats and refined carbohydrates, as well as to genetic factors and aging.

### Insulin Binding on Cells

Obesity causes cell membranes to malfunction. Insulin binds to these membranes only half as well as it does in thin people. Because of this, obese people require larger amounts of insulin than thin people do to achieve the same effect. Fasting helps obese people learn how to manage their appetites and lose weight. But more importantly, this discipline reverses the process of damage to the cells and allows insulin to bind on cells in a more normal way. This helps to bring the diabetes under control. Fasting helps to increase insulin receptors on the cells.

Fasting can be done easily by omitting supper on day one and all meals on day two. On day three, the fast can be broken by eating one-quarter the size of the usual breakfast, one-half the usual lunch and no supper. On day four, three-quarters of the usual breakfast can be eaten. Lunch on day four will be the first full meal after the fast.

## Several Studies of Interest

### Pima Indians

A group of Pima Indians with impaired glucose tolerance was studied. Pima's are noted for their high incidence of obesity and NIDDM. Researchers found increased insulin levels, and a normal pancreatic response to the presence of high levels of sugar in the blood. This indicated that insulin resistance, rather than a failure to produce insulin, was operative in this group. Insulin resistance means the pancreas is producing an ample quantity of insulin, possibly even a surplus quantity, but the body cells are ignoring it. The reason this happens in Type II diabetics is be-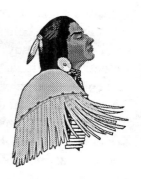cause their cells do not possess adequate numbers of insulin receptors to utilize the insulin which the pancreas is producing to excess.[7]

Factors known to reduce the number of insulin receptors are overeating, use of alcohol and sugar, being overweight, eating too great a variety of food at one meal, eating highly refined or concentrated foods in large quantities, eating between meals, late night meals and the use of meat, milk, eggs and cheese. Inactivity and certain drugs may also reduce insulin receptors. These drugs include oral contraceptives, hormones such as growth hormones, cortisone types of drugs and estrogen.

When the Pimas were living in their natural habitat, diabetes was unknown among them. But when they were sent to reservations and began to adapt to the white man's lifestyle and food, 60-70% of the adults became overweight and 50% became diabetic.

Insulin resistance was worsened by obesity. The study report commented, "Glucose itself can have adverse effects on the pancreas. For example, experimental hyperglycemia (high blood sugar) can worsen abnormalities of pancreatic functions in humans.... It seems ...possible that the beta cells of all persons are susceptible to the 'glucose toxicity....'"[8] In other words, the higher the blood level of glucose, the more damage will be done to organs and tissues, whether or not there is a family history of diabetes.

This is important information for non-diabetics. No person

should feel at liberty to over-indulge in sugar, as it will endanger body cells.

In another study, 16 patients with NIDDM and 14 non-diabetics were matched for age, sex and obesity. Both patients and controls secreted insulin in discrete pulses: normals every 13-14 minutes, but diabetics were irregular and erratic.[9]

In a third study, ten relatives of patients with NIDDM were selected because of mild glucose intolerance and obesity. Average fasting blood sugars for the relatives was 97mg%; for controls, it was 79mg%. Essentially normal production of insulin was found in both groups, but the relatives had lost the 12-14 minute pulsations. The authors state, "It is conceivable that even minor elevations of the plasma glucose level may affect insulin response." They also state, "The pulsatile delivery of insulin may have a physiologic effect on the maintenance of the sensitivity of target tissue." "A plausible suggestion is that abnormal pulsations in the timing of insulin secretion is an early feature in the evolution of NIDDM."[10] It has been found that when excess weight is shed, many patients will regain insulin sensitivity. Eating on an irregular schedule or between meals, may upset the regular pulsatile character of insulin secretion.

## Of Very Special Interest

The following studies are of special interest because for the first time researchers are looking at the possibility that excess sugar itself may be toxic to the pancreas and have an important role in causing diabetes. All people who have a family history of diabetes need to take special note of this possibility. Sugar should be regarded with great suspicion and handled like the highly concentrated substance it is being discovered to be. Also, this is the first time we have seen in print the suggestion that "even minor elevations of plasma glucose levels may affect insulin response." These "minor elevations" averaged only 97 mg, well in the "normal" range by most laboratory reckoning.

These things should be remembered the next time you are thinking about eating your usual dessert of ice cream and cake, because these sweets may be affecting you in more ways than you are aware. Sugary sweets do more damage to our bodies than causing cavities and adding extra weight.

It is also interesting to note what happens when "hyperalimentation" is recommended as a treatment for people who are starving to death. Hyperalimentation is the method of feeding a high glucose (sugar) solution to people who must be artificially fed. In many cases, insulin has to be given to these patients also, because they begin to have pancreatic failure from the high levels of sugar they are ingesting. In some instances, susceptible people who have had hyperalimentation, may develop diabetes.

These findings underscore the long-held contention of the authors, that patients with blood sugars on the upper side of normal should be studied carefully for glucose intolerance or early NIDDM. The effect of mi-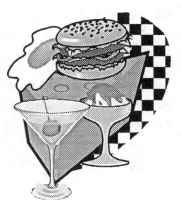nor elevations of blood sugar on the pulsatile secretion of insulin, and the strong suggestion that the pulsatile secretion is essential to maintain normal sensitivity of tissues, has enormous implications regarding regularity of eating, eating between meals, overeating and the gross overuse of sweet foods and drinks.

### Yemini Jews

Studies on the incidence of Type II diabetes in the Yemeni Jews were also done. The ancestral home of these people was the Yemen, where the most common work was that of herding. Their lifestyle included maintaining a simple diet, keeping a regular schedule of life activities and eating almost no refined sugars. There were no cases of diabetes among them. Because of the conflicts between the Arabs and the Jews, the Yemenis had to leave their homeland and move to Israel. In order to adapt to a different society they had to make certain significant

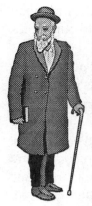

changes in their lifestyle. The main changes were an increase in sugar consumption and a decrease in exercise, both of which led to heavier body weights. After 20 years of living in their new environment with these changes, one out of every five Yemenites over the age of 30 is diabetic. This works out to 20% of their population.

Tests done with laboratory animals put on the "Western diet" for two months revealed that the animals began to develop diabetes. In another group of laboratory animals fed the no-sugar diet of the Yemenites, no diabetes was found, and the animals remained normal.

### Noru

Another investigation was made on an island in the Pacific called Noru. Since World War II, the people have become quite wealthy due to the sale of phosphates, which are abundant on their island. There is one car and one motor bike for every four individuals. They no longer grow any food of their own, but instead import nearly all Western foods. The average daily food intake is 6,100 calories. In the United States the average caloric intake is 2,500. On Noru, 40% of the people have become diabetic.

### Eskimos

A study was also done by Dr. Otto Schaefer, a specialist in

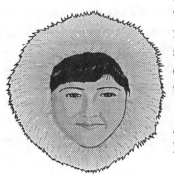

internal medicine, who lived and worked as a physician in the Arctic for 20 years. During the time he spent in his field work he observed drastic changes in the disease patterns of the Eskimos.

In 1959, the Eskimos were ingesting 26 pounds of sugar per person each year. This is a small amount in comparison with the average American's consumption of 130 pounds each year. The Eskimo's 26 pounds of sugar represented 18% of their total carbohydrate intake. 82% of their carbohydrates came from unrefined cereals, flours and starchy foods.

In 1967, only eight years later, the Eskimos were taking in 104.2 pounds of sugar per person each year. This represented 44% of their total carbohydrate intake. Carbohydrates from unrefined foods had dropped to 55%. Dr. Schaefer commented, "The dietary changes seen in the Eskimos parallel those seen in the Western diet over the past 100 years, but they occurred in the Eskimos in eight years."

These changes were due to several factors. The Alcan Highway had opened up and brought more traffic into the Eskimo territory. Other influences were the many air bases built over Alaska and Canada, which brought the Western lifestyle, including an appetite for sweets, to the Eskimos. Dr. Schaefer remarked, "Eskimos seem to have an insatiable desire for candies, sweet cakes and sweet drinks; the mothers often put nipples on pop bottles and the babies suck on them throughout the day."

Dr. Schaefer now found problems among the Eskimos that had not been seen prior to these dietary changes. He noticed the following:

1. Dental decay. This had been nearly unknown among the Eskimos. Photos showed older Eskimos with beautiful, white teeth, and younger Eskimos with missing teeth and blackened stubs which needed to be pulled. Even children needed to have their baby teeth removed. When their permanent teeth came in, these too were decayed and many times had to be extracted.

2. Growth acceleration. The Eskimos were getting heavier and taller. In the past, growth acceleration had been noted among other people after they migrated to the United States or other Western countries from so-called, "developing nations." Experts

claimed that the reason for this increase in weight and height was the introduction of more protein into the diet. But the Eskimos' natural diet has one of the highest percentages of protein consumption in the world. They lived mostly on fat and meat such as seal blubber, fish and polar bear meat, because their native climate inside the arctic circle is not warm enough to grow many vegetables. The only change in their diet was the sudden large intake of refined

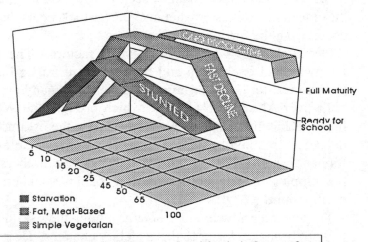

On a high fat, meat-based diet, children are usually ready for school at five years. On a vegetarian diet, children are not ready for school until six to nine years. Both reach full maturity, the fat diet group at around 10-13 years, the vegetarian group from 14-18 years (children on a starvation diet never reach full maturity). But the fat diet group begins dying of degenerative diseases at age 45, and most are dead by age 65. The vegetarian group do not begin to die of degenerative disease until age 70, and most are dead by 100. The stunted group are variable in their death rates.

carbohydrates.

Not only were they getting heavier and taller, but they were going through puberty earlier. Forty years ago, the average Eskimo girl would go through puberty at 18 or 19 years of age. The age of puberty had dropped to 11 years, and has continued to drop back further with each decade. Dr. Schaefer believed the sugar explosion affected the entire endocrine system including the thyroid, growth hormone, and the gonadal hormones of men and women, which caused earlier maturation. He also noted that early menarche was due to a diet of store-bought foods, particularly manufactured foods with a high-content of refined sugar and fat, as opposed to the original native diet. Studies show that the earlier one goes through puberty, the earlier one dies. Also, an 11 year-old child who has reached reproductive maturity must face many social problems. He or she would not have these particular problems if maturity had been delayed until the late teens. School dropouts, the "generation gap," illegal drug use and many other social ills may be traceable to diet in a large percentage of cases.

3. Diabetes. In 1971, there were three times as many cases in Alaska and Greenland than there were in 1961. Now there are more diabetics in one certain group of Eskimos, than there were in all the Eskimos of Canada just a few years ago. Diabetic complications such as heart disease, atherosclerosis, appendicitis, tonsillitis, circulatory disease, cataracts and kidney failure are now beginning to be seen. These complications usually lag 10-20 years after diagnosis.

4. Gall bladder disease. This was a surprise to Dr. Schaefer because it had been assumed that fats played a large role in this problem. It was believed the Eskimos had a genetic ability to handle fat better than Westerners. Prior to 1950, gall bladder disease was unknown among the Eskimos, although 60% of their calories came from fat. This percentage is higher than the 40-45% of calories from fat that is eaten in the standard diet in the lower 48 states. Now the most common operation done in Eskimo hospitals is for removal of the gall bladder due to disease and stones! This is recognized to be due to adding sugar to an already high-fat diet.

5. Obesity and high cholesterol. Dr. Schaefer also noticed several other conditions begin to emerge. Elevated blood fats and obesity were suddenly seen, especially among the urbanized, inactive Eskimos.
6. Skin problems. These people had previously been known for their smooth, clear skin, but now the young people were plagued with acne. The Eskimos themselves are now starting to believe there is something about their diet that is bringing on these "new" problems.

All of the people in the above studies - the Noru Islanders, Pima Indians, Yemeni Jews and the Eskimos - are susceptible to inbreeding. Inbreeding tends to multiply genetic abnormalities and can predispose people to a greater risk for diabetes, as well as other diseases. But it has also been shown that if these people do not become overweight, they generally do not develop diabetes.

These studies clearly point to a link between the Western lifestyle and diabetes. With this information in mind, we need to carefully consider our own lifestyles and habits, and honestly ask ourselves if we are willing to make the changes that will lead to an improved quality of life.

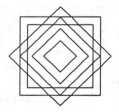

# CHAPTER THREE

# Insulin Resistance

## INSULIN RESISTANCE

For years we have understood that people with Type II 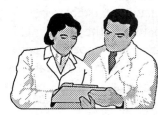 diabetes (NIDDM) were producing high levels of insulin but their cells refused to use it. It is recognized that in order for insulin to be used by body cells it must be taken up by the cell membranes at sites called insulin receptors. Somehow these sites stop functioning well when one overeats or inherits a certain gene. The body tries to overcome the failure of the insulin receptor sites by overproducing insulin to try and force it into the cells with its load of sugar.

Insulin receptors are tiny, submicroscopic receptors on cells. They act as "docking stations" for insulin. The insulin molecule attaches to them and is taken into the cell, where it acts to catalyze the oxidation (speed up the transformation) of glucose into ATP (energy). One-third of glucose is oxidized, and the other two-thirds is converted into glycogen (compressed sugar molecules for storage), which is stored in the liver and muscles until it is needed to be broken down and converted into energy. It seems that during the process of synthesizing the glycogen, a metabolic abnormality occurs in susceptible patients. This abnormality is identical to that seen in most patients with high blood pressure, coronary heart disease and Type II diabetes!

Insulin resistance is defined as a disorder in which cells respond sluggishly to insulin. It is estimated that up to 25% of people in America who are not overweight, inherit or acquire insulin resistance, which compels their pancreas to turn out extra insulin to keep their blood sugar levels normal. The longstanding elevation of insulin in the blood damages the heart and arteries in an unknown process which results in atherosclerosis (hardening of the arteries). Most Type II diabetics are insulin resistant.

There are only two mechanisms to explain why a person becomes diabetic--not enough insulin produced, or the body cells are not responding to the insulin that is produced. The normal person has about ten microunits per milliliter of insulin in the blood while fasting. When insulin resistant, a person may have 30 or more microunits of insulin in the blood. This extra insulin keeps the blood sugar inside the normal range, but at a penalty of damage to the heart. Both Type II diabetes and obesity are usually insulin resistant states. Insulin measured at any one of several levels--fasting, one-hour or two-hour insulin levels--will predict who will have myocardial infarctions in five to ten years. If the insulin level is up, expect trouble unless corrective measures are taken.

Apparently, both a predisposing type of genetics and the presence of an improper diet combine to cause diabetes. People with a family history of diabetes should never use cow's milk or introduce solid food to infants before the age of six months and preferably not before 10-12 months. Several studies have shown that drinking cow's milk before the age of six months increases the likelihood the child will subsequently develop diabetes, buth Type I and II. Even small quantities of skim milk (less than 1% of the diet!) can encourage the development of diabetes at a later time.[11]

Risk factors that appear together as a group and are associated with diabetes, have been collectively named the Insulin Resistance Syndrome, Syndrome X, or Hyperinsulinism. The increased risks include hypertension, upper body (abdominal) obesity, insulin resistance, dyslipidemia characterized by low HDL cholesterol (the good cholesterol) and high triglycerides.

We can begin to understand the widespread development of these disorders when we recognize that the three most common metabolic problems seen in 80% of the people who visit a doctor's office are:

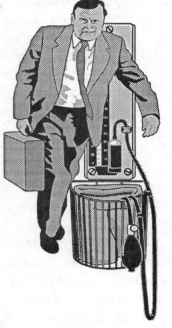

1. *Obesity*: One out of three people are at least 30 pounds overweight
2. *Type II diabetes*: 5-15% of our population
3. *High blood pressure*: One out of five people

These conditions which occur together as a syndrome, accelerate in intensity as people get older. As people age, they become less responsive to insulin. By age 70, one out of four people is diabetic; one out of two is obese; and one out of two has hypertension. This is not a chance association. It now appears to be characteristic of the Insulin Resistance Syndrome. Arteriosclerotic cardiovascular disease (especially coronary heart disease) and abnormal blood fats (low HDL cholesterol and high triglycerides) are also very commonly associated.

## *Causes of Insulin Resistance*

1. There are two ways to become insulin resistant - through **genetics** and/or **overeating**. Usually both factors are present. When insulin levels are high, the insulin directly damages blood vessels to promote atherosclerosis, the most common form of hardening of the arteries.
2. As we **age** we become more and more insulin resis-

tant, probably from a lifetime of overeating. In hypertensives there is a recognized accelerated rate of atherosclerosis.

3. Overeating in diabetic mice caused elevation of insulin levels much higher than overeating in nondiabetic mice of the same age after both groups were given a glucose load.[12]

4. **Chromium**, a mineral known to be active in pancreatic function, has been shown to improve the efficiency of insulin and the blood fat (cholesterol and triglycerides) levels when it is administered as a supplement. It works best if chromium is united to nicotinic acid (vitamin B-3) to make a complex. It is believed by some that chromium deficiency or imbalance may be a factor in the production of insulin resistance.[13]

## Physiology of Insulin Resistance

1. Skeletal muscle has been implicated as the major site of insulin resistance.[14]

2. A normal person's body will store two-thirds of his glucose after a meal and oxidize one-third. In diabetics, hypertensives and coronary patients, there is a defect in the glycogen synthetic pathway.

3. It was found that chiroinositol, a sugar closely related to glucose, was deficient in insulin resistant rats and monkeys. [15]

## Relation of Insulin Resistance to High Blood Pressure

It has been demonstrated that patients with hypertension showed decreased insulin sensitivity and increased insulin secretion.[16] As stated earlier, insulin resistant people have increased coronary heart disease risks,

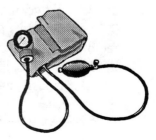

high blood pressure, elevated triglycerides and decreased HDL's.

How does elevated blood insulin cause disturbances in cholesterol and triglyceride levels? The liver makes VLDL (very low density lipoprotein-a blood fat), the synthesis of which is controlled by insulin! Generally we think of insulin only in terms of glucose control, not fat production. Raise insulin and more VLDL is produced. When VLDL is hydrolyzed (decomposition due to incorporation of water) it becomes IDL (intermediate density lipoprotein), one of the most atherogenic (blood vessel damaging) particles found in the body. We can see that one possible cause of elevated blood cholesterol is the production of too much insulin. When blood sugar is even slightly elevated, it may stimulate cholesterol production!

IDL is in high concentration in all insulin resistant states. It is then converted to LDL (low density lipoprotein), leaving a pure cholesterol core and pure apo-B-100. These lipids (blood fats) are all fractions of the fat-protein-cholesterol complex, and are potentially damaging to arteries. High blood insulin causes this cascade of lipid disturbances commonly seen in diabetes and obesity with hypertension.

Since the enzyme, lipoprotein lipase, doesn't work in insulin

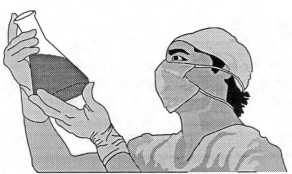

resistance, HDL (high density lipoprotein - the good cholesterol), which is formed when lipoprotein lipase hydrolyzes VLDL to IDL, is going to be low. The major lipid disturbance in Type II diabetics is not so much a high total blood cholesterol as it is a *decrease* in HDL and an *increase* in triglycerides. These are the two major fat disturbances most related to high blood insulin levels and they are very damaging to the arteries.

Insulin resistance (hyperinsulinism-insulin level is high but cells still don't use sugar properly) results in high blood pressure through the following steps: It takes about three days to recover from the effects of eight to ten hours of elevated insulin levels. These levels occur when one indulges in things like overeating birthday cake or eating between meals. These splurges can result in a 4.5-6.5 pound weight gain of fluid in some people. Excess insulin also affects the kidneys to enhance sodium reabsorption by cells and it may take a number of days to eliminate the excess sodium/fluid. Sodium inside the cells increases and this sensitizes smooth muscle cells in blood vessels to the effect of angiotensin II, from the kidneys, and norepinephrine, from the adrenals (sympathetic nervous system pressor-high pressure-hormones). These two hormones are designed to raise blood pressure during stress. High insulin levels are perceived by the body as very stressful.

Insulin stimulates proliferation of smooth muscle cells in blood vessels and stimulates production of connective tissue. Lipids and cholesterol are deposited into the smooth muscle cells and become part of the fatty plaque process that narrows the blood vessels, promoting both heart attacks and high blood pressure.

Insulin affects sodium pumps in cell membranes which increase the flow of sodium into cells, causing the cells to become vasospastic (going into a cramp). Insulin also affects calcium transport into cells and forces excess calcium into cells. Too much calcium then stimulates vasospasm and causes hypertension. Vasospasm and hypertension are two typical characteristics of individuals with increased intracellular sodium and intracellular calcium. Increased insulin is capable of causing both!

Adenosine triphosphate (ATP-the energy molecule) may become deficient in insulin resistance, since glucose is not converted to energy as efficiently. An energy-deficient muscle cell is also a vasospastic cell; spasm of the smooth muscle cells in the blood vessels raises blood pressure.

For the past 35 years, these conditions have been the rationale for the use of diuretic drugs to reduce sodium in order to decrease high blood pressure. But while they may decrease blood pressure, it has become apparent that diuretics do not lessen the risk of coronary heart disease. In fact, they may even increase the risk, especially when used with the beta-blockers, a type of drug that blocks certain nerve receptors.   T h e s e two classes of drugs have an adverse effect on the insulin sensitivity of muscle cells. They aggravate insulin resistance, and promote blood fat  formation. The detrimental effects outweigh any beneficial effects of lowering blood pressure. Although these facts are well known, these types of drugs are still used frequently by physicians, including cardiologists.

Dr. Norman Kaplan, a distinguished cardiologist, questions the morality of the 20% increase in use of these drugs since reports of their dangers started being published.  In response to these reports, the drug companies stepped up their advertising in hopes of nullifying this financially damaging information. This advertising resulted in the increased use of these drugs.

## *The Sympathetic Nervous System, High Blood Pressure and Insulin Resistance*

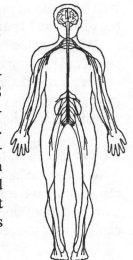

Excess insulin also activates the sympathetic nervous system (SNS).  The SNS mediates the link between increased insulin in the blood and essential hypertension. This is caused by an increase in norepinephrine in the blood. Injecting insulin in the vein of a patient's forearm caused norepinephrine release into the forearm at a threefold greater amount in hypertensives than in normal controls.[17]

Fasting or caloric restriction suppresses SNS activity, while overfeeding stimulates it. Carbohydrates and fats both stimulate SNS activity, even when total caloric intake is not increased. This operates through the hypothalamus in the brain. A drop in glucose and insulin (as in fasting) decreases insulin-mediated uptake in the hypothalamus and decreases activity of the SNS. Conversely, an increase in either glucose or insulin increases uptake and stimulates the SNS. "Insulin is thus a signal that permits the brain to assess nutritional status and adjust sympathetic outflow accordingly."[18]

Lewis Landsberg, author of *Insulin Resistance, Energy Balancing and Sympathetic Nervous System Activity,*[19] considers that insulin resistance in the obese is a compensatory mechanism to increase the metabolic rate, which in turn helps to stabilize body weight and help prevent further obesity.

This may also be what happens in non-obese hypertensives who are insulin resistant. They may have well-developed mechanisms that will increase energy expenditure to resist weight gain and maintain energy balance, even when they increase their calorie intake. Instead of overweight, they develop high insulin levels and SNS stimulation, which induce high blood pressure. In one study it was found that lean people with high blood pressure were much more likely to become obese over an 11 year follow-up, than were non-hypertensives.

Oxidizing glucose in the cell generates ATP. But if a muscle cell is not binding insulin and becomes energy-deficient, that cell becomes vasospastic. Cells found in the smooth muscles in blood vessels can become insulin resistant, causing the vasospasm which produces hypertension.

### Relation of Insulin Resistance to Cancer

Women who have increased insulin in the blood with insulin resistance have a significantly higher risk of breast cancer independent of body weight or fat distribution.[20] Pancreatic cancer has also been associated with insulin resistance.[21], [22], [23]

## *Relation of Insulin Resistance to Diabetes*

Diabetics and the obese are both insulin resistant, but obese nondiabetics have a glucose curve like normals. Their blood sugar is maintained at a normal level by the production of two and a half to three times greater amounts of insulin than that produced by lean nondiabetics. It can be predicted by observing levels of insulin in children three years of age, which ones will develop diabetes later in life. Those with higher levels of insulin are more likely to develop diabetes.

If for any reason the beta cells of the pancreas slightly reduce the amount of insulin produced, the obese person will become diabetic, since the pancreas was already overproducing insulin to compensate for insulin resistance. Even a slight reduction in insulin throws the person into diabetes.

## *Effects on The Kidneys*

As described earlier, insulin has a hormone effect that causes the kidneys to hold onto sodium. This is why Christmas holiday sweets can cause sodium retention and the gaining of five to six pounds of weight every week during the "sweets 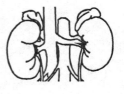 season." This process increases sodium concentration in smooth muscle cells of blood vessels. There, the sodium sensitizes those cells to the pressor effects of the hormones angiotensin II and norepinephrine, which cause narrowing of blood vessels and raises blood pressure.

Activation of the sympathetic nervous system also occurs with increased circulating norepinephrine. As insulin goes up, norepinephrine goes up. When the "fight or flight" portion of the nervous system is activated, a secondary insulin resistance follows creating a vicious circle.

## *Treatment*

Losing weight and increasing physical exercise can both help the body use insulin more efficiently.[24]

Exercise is a known treatment for insulin resistance. Perhaps the reason high blood pressure, cancer, diabetes and heart disease are all so successfully treated with exercise is the 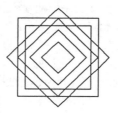 primary benefit exercise gives in decreasing insulin resistance.

Fasting is another major treatment modality for insulin resistance. We have been aware for years that diabetes is profoundly benefited by fasting. The reason for this is that fasting improves insulin sensitivity.[25]

Other important aspects of treatment include the use of foods high in magnesium, vanadium and chromium. See Chapter Eleven for other essential nutrients in the treatment of insulin resistance, and the foods known to highest in these nutrients.

# CHAPTER FOUR

# *General Facts About Diabetes And The Physiology Involved*

The use of sugar in the United States now amounts to 130-150 pounds per person per year; more than one-third of a pound per day. This means each person is taking over one cup of sugar every day. Even as early as 1900, the average person suspected we were using far too much sugar at only 15 pounds per person per year. It was believed even then, that sugar was the cause of certain diseases.

By 1930, at about 85 pounds per person per year, it was obvious to the physicians of that day that the heavy sugar consumption caused the great increase in diabetes since 1900. Now we recognize not only damage to the teeth (the number of new caries developed per year is directly proportional to the number of times per day a child eats something sweet), but also damage to the heart and arteries, emotional problems from altered brain metabolism and damage to the immune mechanism which causes one to be less able to ward off infections, including infections by cancer viruses. This is one reason diabetics are more likely to develop cancer than are non-diabetics. Researchers have recently found a quintuplet of diseases that travel together: diabetes, altered blood fats (cholesterol and triglycerides), cancer, high blood pressure and abdominal obesity.

## *Diabetes Facts And Figures*

The incidence rate of **diabetes in Michigan children** doubled between 1959 and 1972.[26] This reflects a general "diabetes explosion" which has been going on for many decades.

**Juvenile onset type diabetes** is apparently inherited by a recessive gene which affects about half its carriers. Adult onset diabetes is apparently a dominant genetic disorder, inherited via a single dominant gene, possibly linked to the HLA (human-leukocyte-antigen) system.[27,28]

**Urine glucose** is lowered by adding guar gum, a gel made up of leguminous fiber, to the diet of diabetics. Fiber ties up excessive glucose and makes the glucose unavailable to the blood.[29]

The risk of insulin-dependent-diabetes (IDDM) is greater in **very young mothers** than it is in older mothers.[30] Very young diabetic women should probably delay having children until they are over 25 or 30 years of age.

Statistically the **fetal death rate** is 10.4 times higher with

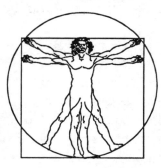

diabetic than non-diabetic pregnancies. After birth, the infants of diabetic mothers have a 5.5 times higher mortality rate during the first six months of life. This indicates that the metabolic and immune functions are weaker in diabetic mothers; a weakness that is then passed on to their offspring.

More **unborn infants** of diabetic mothers die in each period of pregnancy; the first 3 months, second 3 months, last 3 months, during labor and in every birthweight category.[31]

**Congenital malformations** and developmental problems during the first five years of life are more common in infants born to diabetic mothers, than to those infants born to non-diabetic mothers. This is particularly true if the baby is born smaller than would be expected for the length of the pregnancy.

A **low infant birthweight** and the presence of acetone in the mother's urine during pregnancy are both associated with adverse effects on the intelligence of the offspring for at least the first five years of life.[32]

**Inactivity, oral contraceptives and diuretics** can cause glucose intolerance.

An early sign of **pancreatic cancer** is a high fasting blood sugar level.[33]

**Insulin release** from the pancreas into the blood occurs as a direct response to a rising blood sugar level. Nerve impulses through a cranial nerve called the vagus nerve, also play a role in insulin regulation. High levels of insulin increase the risk of high blood pressure and coronary heart disease, as discussed earlier.

**Insulin,** which keeps blood sugar from going too high, originates in the pancreas from the beta cells. **Glucagon** which keeps blood sugar from going too low, originates in the alpha cells of the pancreas. Glucagon contains the amino acids methionine and tryptophane, and has an effect similar to adrenalin on the release mechanism of blood sugar. Growth hormone from the pituitary stimulates normal alpha cell production of glucagon. Growth hormone is produced in adults only during exercise in the daytime and only during sleep at night, mainly before midnight. This is a good reason to go to bed early.

**Prediabetic mothers** who overeat will have an overproduction of growth hormone. The heavy birth weights of their babies are related to this increased growth hormone in the mother. Diabetic children tend to be tall because of this mechanism. Too much food causes the pituitary to overproduce growth hormone, which indirectly raises insulin levels, increasing one's risk of high blood pressure. But normal food intake and abundant sleep normalize the output of growth hormone.

In diabetes, **energy production** via glucose oxidation, protein synthesis, wound healing, fatty acid synthesis, as well as storage of glycogen, are all impaired. The oxidation of fructose in order to make energy is not impaired in the diabetic. Fructose is a simple sugar generally present in fruits. Fruits may be eaten relatively freely by Type II diabetics as a general rule. However, if fructose is isolated from fruit and used by diabetics, it will impair the function of insulin, making transport of nutrients more difficult. Glucose, also a simple sugar, is highest in grains and starchy vegetables.

For reasons not yet clear to geneticists, our population has become **genetically prone** to developing diabetes. It is possible that our genes have undergone a mutation, similar to what happens to certain insects when they are continuously exposed to pesticides, or many other chemicals. Perhaps our genes have been continuously exposed to harmful chemicals, drugs and refined nutrients until they have "mutated" into a weaker form and are passed to offspring in this state. However, a genetically prone person can prevent the onset of diabetes by cutting down on total food consumption, especially of refined sugars, including sucrose, glucose, and fructose, to 5% of the total carbohydrate intake, instead of the 50% average in Western diets. The sugars found in fruits, vegetables, whole grains and nuts are in their naturally occurring form and are combined with other substances in these foods to help the body properly utilize these sugars.

**Only 13% of diabetics** are instructed by their physicians on diet. Yet, perfect control of the nutrition of the diabetic remains the primary way of treating diabetes. Green vegetables are especially good foods for diabetics. The diabetic should be **taught to eat** as little as possible; only enough to maintain ideal weight.

Intermittent **24 hour fasting** has been very beneficial in reducing the amount of sugar in the urine. (See the method for fasting in Chapter Ten.)

Many European investigators have stated that diabetics need to eat **complex carbohydrates** rather than refined foods such as sugar, honey, fats, starch, white flour and white rice. The long-practiced and time-honored American method of treating diabetes, which had been used until recently, featured a diet high in fats and proteins and low in complex carbohydrates. But meats, milk, cheeses, eggs, free fats and too many nuts or meat substitutes, are not helpful to the person suffering with diabetes. Diabetics manage best on a completely vegetarian diet composed of fruits, vegetables, whole grains and a few nuts and seeds. The virtues of potatoes and whole grain rice and cereals, as well as complex carbohydrates, should be emphasized in the diet.

A diabetic who does not take insulin does not need to eat a certain prescribed **number of meals** per day. A prescription for three or four meals per day, at set times, and the use of a measured calorie diet is only necessary for the long-acting insulin user whose insulin has fixed times of peak activity to coincide with usual mealtimes. But the ideal meal pattern for a non-insulin-using diabetic, is to eat a satisfying breakfast and lunch but no supper or snacks. This increases insulin binding to the cells. (See section on insulin-binding in Chapter Three)

Generally for diabetics, **1200-1500 calories per day** are sufficient if the work is sedentary. The inhabitants of Hunza, who are very active farmers, generally eat between 1500 and 1735 calories per day. Most of us eat far too much. Diabetics will manage best on a very spare diet.

Since **most Americans** have at least some tendency towards diabetes, major reforms are needed in diet and education. This type of education should begin in kindergarten or even earlier.

**Coffee** has been found to be harmful to diabetics and to potential diabetics. Higher blood sugar levels have been recorded in diabetics at 30, 60 and 90 minutes following test meals when coffee was added. Individuals with and without coronary disease have been tested after drinking coffee. It was found that **both groups had four to five times more free-fatty acids in their blood after drinking black coffee, than after drinking decaffeinated coffee.** This is important in relation to diabetes, because diabetics are more prone than others to develop coronary disease and high blood pressure. Decaffeinated coffee is also harmful because of the many other detrimental substances in the brown drinks. We recommend that all forms of coffee and its brown drink and food relatives, like tea and chocolate, be removed from the diabetic's diet.

**High doses of insulin,** administered by injections, are linked to development of lipid (fat) disorders. An inverse relationship exists between insulin doses and high density lipoproteins (HDL- the good cholesterol), the substance which transports fats out of the tissues. This suggests that increasing amounts of insulin hinders HDL's ability to remove adequate quantities of cholesterol.[34] Overeating, or eating a sweet dessert and attempting to cover the indulgence with more insulin, is a very unwise practice. Not only does it make you lose control of your appetite, but it endangers both your heart and your arteries.

The use of **too much insulin** also causes the Somogyi effect, or rebound elevation of blood sugar after a period of low blood sugar. This occurs when the physician or the diabetic patient become concerned because the blood sugar climbed to a high level and sugar spilled in the urine. Even though an adequate quantity of insulin, or possibly even too much was already being taken, the insulin dosage is increased. The extra insulin results in another very low blood sugar level and another very high rebound. Again the poor diabetic spills sugar in the urine when the blood sugar was at its peak. The physician may mistakenly believe the patient needs further increases in the insulin dosage. Finally the patient begins to have alternating bouts of insulin reactions and extremely high blood sugar levels.[35] Such a diabetic may be labeled a "brittle diabetic" who is "hard to control." This is not an accurate diagnosis. Adjustment downward of the insulin dosage and careful dietary management are usually all that is required to convert brittle diabetes into controlled diabetes.

An **epidemic of certain viral diseases**, like mumps, will be followed years later by an outbreak of Type I diabetes. As early as 1864, there was a hypothesis linking juvenile diabetes with mumps virus.

Beta cells produce insulin and their loss results in reduced ability to handle not only **sugar**, but also **protein and fat**. Type I diabetes is the result of this loss. Specific strains of mumps viruses attach to the beta cells of the pancreas.[36] The virus then appears to destroy the beta cells.[37] **Other diseases** that may precede diabetes are infectious hepatitis and infectious mononucleosis. Coxsackie viruses and encephalomyocarditis viruses have been followed by diabetes in mice.[38] Coxsackie B-2 virus is capable of attacking the pancreas of children and causing juvenile onset diabetes.[39]

**Infections before birth** with German measles, mumps and other viruses may cause some cases of diabetes. Prenatal infections with German measles virus (rubella) has been proven to be associated with diabetes appearing later in life. Like certain other viruses, the German measles virus is capable of causing both an immediate rash, fever, sore throat, etc., and a slow acting effect resulting in degeneration of the pancreatic islet cells.

The **occurrence of both mumps and diabetes** has 3 irregular cycles, each lasting seven years. There is a four year time lag between these cycles at which time the pancreas may degenerate after being infected by the mumps virus. Diabetes may result from an autoimmune response to "slow viruses" such as the mumps virus. "Fast viruses" are those like the cold virus, which strike and are immediately followed by a disease from which one recovers within a few days or weeks. A slow virus may cause one disease immediately (such as chicken pox), and years later another disease appears (such as shingles). Both the chicken pox and the shingles were caused by the same virus. With Type I diabetes, the virus first caused mumps and later caused diabetes after autoimmune damage to the beta cells of the pancreas.

A group of Australian doctors studied 45 men and women who had been infected with **German measles** virus prenatally. Each of the 45 people studied, had suffered one or more of the classical types of rubella damage since birth such as deafness, eye problems, heart damage or central nervous system damage. 80% developed diabetes in early childhood, while the remaining 20% (nine out of the 45) developed the disease in their twenties. The rubella virus persisted in the congenitally infected human pancreas for months or even years.

Many cases of **adult onset type of diabetes** are now turning up in children. Most of these children are physically inactive, overweight, they eat a diet that is too rich and they have irregular eating patterns--eating at any time of the day or night and eating an improper choice of foods. These young diabetics can be treated with diet alone.

The use of **oral antidiabetic medicines** for children, such as Sulfonylureas, DiaBeta, Diabanese, Glucotrol, Micronase, Orinase and Tolinase, has been criticized because of the toxic effects of these drugs. Patients treated for five to eight years with diet and Tolbutamide, had a rate of cardiovascular mortality two and one-half times higher than the rate of patients treated with diet alone.[40] Thickening of the lining cells of small blood vessels, severe hypoglycemia, jaundice, nausea, heartburn, skin rashes, severe blood cell depletion and other problems have all been noted in children taking oral antidiabetic drugs. There is also lack of evidence that the children's diabetes is improved in any way. There is no substitute for diet and exercise.

Because of the stress of having high blood sugar, the body develops **metabolic stress** (the condition in which organs are overworked due to an unhealthy lifestyle). Add to this stress the emotional and social turbulence often associated with metabolic problems, and a condition known as stress erythrocytosis may develop. This condition is associated with increased blood viscosity.

**Viscosity is defined** as a flow characteristic of fluids. For example: water and honey are both fluids, but honey has a higher viscosity. When blood has a large quantity of different chemicals dissolved in it, the viscosity is increased, making the blood thicken and become more like honey. Sugar is one of the chemicals which can cause increased blood viscosity. Elevated viscosity of the blood from high blood sugar levels may be a factor in microangiopathy (disease of the smallest arteries).[41],[42] It is now certain that even small increases in blood sugar will damage blood vessels. (See discussion of stress erythrocytosis and a case history in Chapter Two.)

A Scandinavian study showed that **sexual maturity** was achieved at age seventeen in the early half of the nineteenth century. Today we have much earlier sexual maturity in boys as well as girls. This earlier sexual maturity leads to a series of undesirable consequences. Some things attributed to premature sexual maturation include dropping out of school, marrying too young, bearing illegitimate children, entering into crime, gangs, the drug scene and even becoming homosexual.

It has been theorized that homosexuality might be due to the early sexual development of **emotionally and socially immature young people.** Older children are mainly segregated according to sex; girls associate with girls and boys with boys. Both are naive and incapable of developing a mature relationship with the opposite sex. Many times they are frightened to be in the company of the opposite sex and are concerned about what their same sex peers think. If they become sexually mature at this age and begin to seek sexual gratification, the boys may turn to the boys, and the girls to other girls.

**"Better nutrition,"** as defined by many contemporary nutritionists, is behind this early sexual development. But Dr. Otto Schaefer, who conducted the Eskimo studies discussed in Chapter Two, observed that when people **maintain simple diets, early sexual maturity does not occur.** This problem has only surfaced since people have changed from home-grown diets, to store-bought combinations of highly refined foods that are rich in sugar and fat.

## Physiology of The Development of Diabetes

### Pancreatic Products

The pancreas is a unique organ because it is a member of both the endocrine and exocrine systems.

### Enzymes, Exocrine Substances

The exocrine system is made up of organs with internal gland structures, such as the mouth with its salivary glands, the breast with its milk glands and the skin with its sweat glands. This system produces enzymes and delivers them to various locations in the body by means of tubes.

The pancreas produces lipase, amylase and trypsin, powerful enzymes for breaking down fat, carbohydrates and protein, and delivers them to the first part of the small bowel, the duodenum, which is an organ of the digestive tract.

### Hormones, Endocrine Substances

The endocrine system is composed of glands that produce hormones, which go directly into the bloodstream by crossing blood vessel walls, as they course through the gland. There are no tubes (ducts) for distributing hormones. The thyroid, parathyroids, testes, ovaries, adrenals and pituitary are all members of the endocrine system.

The pancreas produces at least two hormones that go directly into the blood. Blood capillaries go through the little structures in the pancreas, called the Islets of Langerhans, to deliver oxygen and nutrients, and as they pass through, they pick up the hormones. The Islets of Langerhans are peculiarly susceptible to damage by certain chemi-

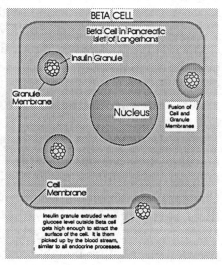

BETA CELL

Beta Cell in Pancreatic Islet of Langerhans

Insulin Granule

Granule Membrane

Nucleus

Fusion of Cell and Granule Membranes

Cell Membrane

Insulin granule extruded when glucose level outside Beta cell gets high enough to attract the surface of the cell. It is then picked up by the blood stream, similar to all endocrine processes.

cal toxins such as coffee and alcohol. In the body, the prime targets of these two substances are the Islets of Langerhans and the brain.

Diabetes is now thought to be a combined alpha and beta cell disorder. The alpha cells of the pancreas produce glucagon which is responsible for keeping the blood sugar from going too low. The beta cells of the pancreas produce insulin which keeps the blood sugar from going too high. Glucagon is also involved in a certain enzymatic process which breaks up glycogen (the storage form of sugar in an animal which corresponds to starch in a plant), the storage form of glucose.

## Pathologic Anatomy and Physiology In Diabetes and The Hypoglycemic Syndrome

Red blood cells are normally quite flexible and easily bent, elongating out of the usual disk shape to slip through vessels with a diameter smaller than their own. Diabetics do not have as much of this folding ability of their red blood cells as non-diabetics, a feature which may contribute to the circulatory abnormalities seen in diabetics and prediabetics. It may be that the stiffened red blood cells actually injure the small capillaries causing an increase in the thickness of the delicate capillary walls.[43] Thickened capillary walls have been found in many patients having diabetes. This process begins very early in life and is an indication that a child has a predisposition to diabetes.

In certain diabetics and hypoglycemics there are abnormal actions of the stomach, one of which is a delay in gastric emptying. In still others, there is such quick emptying it becomes a virtual dumping. In the early phases of the disease, the first condition can be demonstrated as a flat curve in the blood sugar levels of a glucose tolerance test. The latter is evident in reactive hypoglycemia with a very high level in the curve at the 30 minute reading, followed by very low levels at the two-hour reading. Other gastrointestinal abnormalities include diarrhea, constipation, nausea and vomiting.[44]

From the twentieth day of the menstrual cycle onward, there is a slight elevation in blood sugar levels as determined by the glucose tolerance test. This is the time estrogen levels are highest. Glucose tolerance is best at the earliest phase of the cycle and worst in the cycle when estrogen is highest.[45] Estrogen has a diabetogenic effect, which may be one reason why more women tend to have diabetes than men.

## Injury From External Causes

Diabetes is increasing at a rate of six percent a year, and currently affects more than 15 million Americans, either as fullblown diabetes or predisease states. In 1973 it was estimated that 612,000 new cases were identified, an increase of more than 40% over 1965.[46] Approximately 300,000 deaths a year are attributed to diabetes.[47]

### Caffeine Damage To The Pancreas

We have not yet determined the manner in which caffeine damages the Islets of Langerhans. In some way it poisons the system, making it difficult to keep the blood sugar at a proper level. It either stimulates the production of insulin, or inhibits the production of glucagon which causes the blood sugar to drop too low.

### Alcohol Damage To The Pancreas

While both the exocrine and endocrine functions of the pancreas are damaged by alcohol, the endocrine function suffers more acutely. The Islets of Langerhans become smaller and lose many cells. This makes the risk of developing diabetes greater. All forms of pancreatitis are more common in individuals who drink alcohol. It is rare for a person who does not have either acute dehydration or alcoholism to develop pancreatitis. Multiple bouts of pancreatitis can lead to diabetes because of the destruction of the pancreatic tissue.

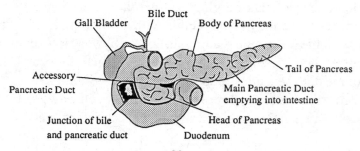

80

Alcohol is also capable of poisoning the system of insulin and glucagon balance. Much of what causes a hangover is the result of low blood sugar. It has been demonstrated that some alcoholics who become mean and abusive while drinking, rather than becoming happy, have severe hypoglycemic reactions to alcohol.

### Spoiled Food Damage

Nitrosamine, a substance that may be formed by spoiled proteins, may be capable of causing diabetes. We should not eat anything that has spoilage in it; not even the smallest taint of spoilage.

### Cow's Milk Damage

A recent report in *TIME* magazine recapped an article which had been written in the *New England Journal of Medicine*, on cow's milk and juvenile diabetes. The *Journal* said that the principal culprit for causing juvenile diabetes may be cow's milk. The article described how doctors at the Hospital for Sick Children in Toronto, found that diabetics have a much higher than normal level of antibodies to a protein in cow's milk called bovine serum albumin. The diabetics' bodies have targeted the protein as an invader to be destroyed. A section of this milk protein is almost identical to a protein on the surface of insulin-producing cells. The doctors theorized that when children are sensitized to milk, they may also be sensitized to their own cells, leading to the destruction of a part of the insulin-producing cells! Many pediatricians are now suggesting that children never need cow's milk, but can be weaned from the breast to the table at one to two years of age. When weaned, a child does not need to start drinking cow's milk.

### Other Causes Of Diabetes

Certain drugs can also cause diabetes. The corticosteroids are recognized as creating conditions within the body leading to the development of diabetes (Cortisone, Prednisone, Ilosone, etc.). Birth control pills can be even more hazardous and conducive to the development of diabetes because of their widespread and long-continued use. Diuretics (Diamox, Lasix, Aldactone, Dyazide, Diuril, Hydrodiuril) may also contribute to high blood sugar because of their dehydrating effect.

As we have seen in this chapter, there can be other physiological reasons, as well as lifestyle causes, that can lead to the onset of diabetes. We have also discussed many different factors involved in the evolution of diabetes. Some of the factors are highly technical, while others are as common as what we eat for breakfast. Hopefully, every reader will have no difficulty in understanding the conclusions drawn. Careful study of these facts and figures and the application of appropriate measures, will result in a reduced risk of developing diabetes and its four traveling companions, hypertension, cancer, heart disease and abdominal obesity, at any age.

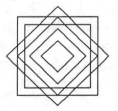

# CHAPTER FIVE

# *Experimental Work*

Studies of native diets as compared to our contemporary diet, and surveys of other factors known to contribute to the onset of diabetes, are only a part of the current diabetic research. Researchers have also been conducting controlled experiments designed to show how different foods affect fat and sugar levels in diabetics and non-diabetics.

## *Lower the Fats and Increase The Fiber*

Dietary fiber can cause a decrease in both cholesterol and blood sugar in Type I and Type II diabetics. Six Type I and eight Type II diabetics were given a ten day weight-maintaining diet of three different types: 1) low carbohydrate-low fiber (42% and 20gm. respectively); 2) high carbohydrate-low fiber (53%, 16gm.); and 3) high carbohydrate-high fiber (53%, 54gm.). The most favorable outcome of the tests revealed that two-hour post-prandial (after meal) blood sugar readings showed a significant decrease in blood sugar and cholesterol only with the high carbohydrate-high fiber diets. Based on these experiments, it could be stated that merely altering the fat or carbohydrate content of the diet may not improve the control of blood sugar or cholesterol unless there is an increase in fiber at the same time.[48]

In practical terms, this means eating with an emphasis on complex carbohydrates as found in fruits, vegetables and whole grains. Use of refined fats such as butter, margarine, mayonnaise, fried foods, salad oils, cooking fats and peanut butter, and refined carbohydrates like white sugar, white rice, white pastas, white bread, all white flour products and alcoholic beverages, must be entirely cut out of the diet for the best results.

In another experiment, a 20gm. fiber diet and a 3gm. fiber diet were given to diabetics for 10 days and the results compared. Total calories, carbohydrates, fat and protein were identical in the two diets. Seven of eight patients on the higher fiber diet showed a lower glucose level.[49]

These studies show that diabetics who are given a fat-free, high-complex-carbohydrate, high-fiber diet, respond well.[50] Patients who use insulin are able to decrease their dosage because of lower glucose levels. Those patients who do not use insulin show a similar improvement in blood glucose levels.[51]     The vegan vegetarian diet, using no animal products (no meat, milk, eggs or cheese), and having the highest fiber content of any diet, is the most beneficial diet for diabetics.

## High Fat, High Protein Not Good

A liberalized carbohydrate intake is now being recommended in the United States, in contrast to the high-fat, high-protein, low carbohydrate intake which was formerly recommended for diabetics. The purpose of this liberalized carbohydrate intake is to help in reducing kidney disease, eye problems, obesity, cancer and high cholesterol and triglyceride levels. These are associated with kidney and liver disease, atherosclerosis and heart and artery disease, which are accompanied by heart attacks and strokes. All are promoted by high fat and protein intakes.[52] Maturity onset diabetes, a form of accelerated aging, is also connected with a high-fat, high-protein, low carbohydrate diet.

Diabetics will show lower fasting and mean serum triglyceride values while on a high carbohydrate diet, rather than on the high fat, high-protein diet which was popularized for so many years by the American Diabetes Association.[53]

## Diabetic Complications

In diabetics, 80% of the deaths are due to blood vessel disease. In non-diabetics, only 40% of the deaths are due to blood vessel disease. Fats and proteins in the diet trigger the development of this disease in both diabetics and non-diabetics.

Adult diabetics in Japan have very little gangrene. It is thought that the high carbohydrate diet consisting mainly of starches from natural sources and not table sugar, is an important factor. Researchers have learned recently that the taking of insulin may also promote atherosclerosis rather than preventing it. Studies showed that injections of large doses of insulin into rats for a period of several weeks caused changes leading to atherosclerosis. (See discussion on Insulin Resistance in Chapter Three.)

Insulin injections should be avoided if possible, but if essential, should be taken in the smallest dose that is reasonable to control the blood sugar. This makes control of diet and other lifestyle factors very important, as blood sugar must not be allowed to run riot.

### Jerusalem Artichokes Good for Diabetics

An experiment was done in which a diabetic patient was given half of his carbohydrates in the form of Jerusalem artichokes, tubers of a plant in the sunflower family. The daily absorption of major nutrients included 50 grams of protein, 40 grams of fat and 205 grams of carbohydrate, with a total energy content of about 1500 calories. On one day the artichokes were replaced with baked potatoes. The patient's urine had been sugar-free for some time on a diet in which artichokes furnished the greater portion of the carbohydrates. The substitution of baked potatoes on one day was accompanied by an increase of urinary nitrogen and the prompt appearance of sugar in the urine, a rise in the blood sugar and an increase in heat production.

The results of the test with the Jerusalem artichokes indicates an interesting finding. When artichokes furnish at least 50% percent of the daily intake of carbohydrates, the body can absorb and utilize the carbohydrates, even if diabetes mellitus is present.[54] Jerusalem artichokes are high in inulin, a complex carbohydrate which seems to be the substance that produces the beneficial effects. Even though potatoes are a very good food, they are not used as well as Jerusalem artichokes by the diabetic.

*Fenugreek Seeds*

A study on the effect of fenugreek seeds on blood glucose, cholesterol and triglyceride levels, showed that when defatted fenugreek seed powder was incorporated into the diet, fasting blood sugar was significantly reduced and the glucose tolerance test readings were improved. 100 grams of fenugreek seed powder (slightly less than one half cup) was divided into two equal doses and served with two daily meals. Total serum cholesterol, LDL, VLDL and triglycerides were also significantly reduced. The HDL cholesterol remained unchanged. The conclusion based on these studies is that fenugreek seeds are useful in the management of Type I diabetes.

*Raw Foods Good*

Plasma glucose levels decreased in both mild and severe diabetics after a raw meal as compared to a cooked meal of the same caloric value. This suggests that a better insulin-glucose relationship is obtained from eating raw foods.[55]

*Onions Good*

The onion has certain components which lower the blood sugar level. Onions may be useful as a blood sugar-lowering agent for diabetics. Interestingly, the blood sugar of normal individuals is not lowered by eating onions.[56]

## Low-Fat Diet

Diets low in fat and high in fiber improve insulin binding, even in patients given a high sucrose dose. The low-fat levels seem to compensate for the excess of sucrose. The conclusion is that the best diet is one 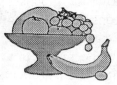 that is low in sucrose and its components, low in fat, and high in fiber.[57]  There is no fiber in meat, milk, eggs or cheese. Unrefined fruits, vegetables and whole grains are high in fiber.

Other studies show low protein levels to be beneficial, also. The ideal diet for the diabetic emphasizes fruit, vegetables and whole grains.  In fruit the sugars are bound to fiber, which enables them to be handled well by the body. Since fat is low in such a diet, it is the most beneficial diet for diabetics.

### Honey and Sugar Similar

While sucrose has many things to condemn it, some individuals believe diabetics can use honey more or less freely. It is a fact, however, that honey is chemically very close to sucrose.  Honey is a disaccharide (meaning two sugars), composed of a solution of glucose and fructose which is slightly acid. By law, commercial honey must be at least 80% sugars.  These concentrated, refined (by the bee) sweeteners deliver a large amount of sugar into the blood stream.  The result is that the blood sugar level rises to a height similar to that found with the use of sucrose.

Studies have been done showing a reduction in the ability of white blood cells to surround, kill or deliver germs to an execution site after an individual has eaten sugar.  Even commercial orange juice with its high sugar content, which may be made up of a certain percentage of refined sugar as well as its own natural sugar, has been shown to reduce this white blood cell capability, or phagocytic index.  The phagocytic index is measured by the number of germs the white blood cells consume in half an hour. When the blood sugar level is high in a diabetic, it reduces the germ-eating capability of white blood cells.  It appears that it is the actual sugar level, and not the chemical make-up of the type of sugar in certain foods, that produces the damage. We can tolerate small amounts of fructose, glucose, sucrose or honey, but never can we safely consume the quantities found in the usual American diets.

## Stress, Adrenalin, and Weight

The production of adrenalin, one of the most powerful lipolytic (fat breakdown) agents we know, increases during stress. Fat then, is broken down faster than it can be stored. This is why some people lose weight when they are under stress, even though their food intake and exercise levels remain the same as the period before the stress began.

In contrast to adrenalin, insulin is the only known lipogenic (fat-building) agent. In some people the mechanism for producing insulin is stronger than the mechanism for producing adrenalin. Their fat storage capabilities exceed their fat breakdown abilities. These people gain weight when under stress. One thing that causes stress is a high blood sugar. Through a complex biochemical mechanism, it causes the release of nor-adrenalin, which increases blood pressure and encourages coronary heart disease and cancer. (See discussion on Insulin Resistance in Chapter Three)

## Other Lipolytic Substances

While adrenalin is the most powerful agent for breaking down fats, there are others such as nor-adrenalin, ACTH, and the glucocorticoids which are the hormones from the adrenal cortex or exterior layer of the adrenal glands (adrenalin comes only from the adrenal medulla or center). Also included are the growth hormone from the pituitary gland and thyroxin from the thyroid. As mentioned earlier, in adults growth hormone is produced only during exercise and sleep mainly before midnight. It is made very poorly or not at all during daytime naps.

## Fasting Helps

Fasting helps obese, Type II diabetics stop injections of insulin. In one study, a seven day food and insulin-free fast, followed by a low calorie diet, was successful in helping 34 out of 37 overweight, diabetic patients, to stop using insulin.[58] Plasma insulin falls in individuals who are starving. This principle can be utilized by fasting patients to give the pancreas a rest.[59] The pancreas will almost always operate better after fasting from one to eight meals. Fasting is a standard treatment for diabetes of the adult onset type-Type II. (See Chapter Ten for the correct method of fasting.) A Type I (juvenile) diabetic should never fast.

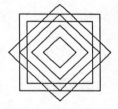

# CHAPTER SIX

# Complications and Treatment of Diabetes

## DIET FACTORS

Diabetologists are now beginning to accept the fact that in countries other than the United States, the treatment for diabetes has been far more fruitful in the long run, than the traditional treatments used by American physicians. The formula that has been more suc-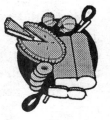cessful has supplied most of a patient's **calorie needs from carbohydrates rather than from fats or proteins**, as doctors in the United States generally advocated. Whole grains, vegetables, fruits and other complex carbohydrates are handled better by diabetics, than animal products and free fats.

It is well known that **free fats** increase the risk of the traveling companion diseases for which diabetics are particularly prone, such as cancer, hardening of the arteries, arthritis, hypertension and overweight. **Animal proteins** and concentrated plant proteins found in substitute meat products, increase the incidence of kidney disease. **White flours, white grains, white breads** and other foods changed from their natural state by mechanical and/or chemical processing and known as refined carbohydrates, accelerate the rate of production of arterial disease and insulin resistance.

Because of these problems, we remove most concentrated foods and all free fats from the diabetic diet at Uchee Pines Institute. Margarine, mayonnaise, fried foods, cooking fats, salad oils, nut butters and dairy products, as well as a large proportion of nuts, seeds and wheat germ are left out of the diet. Food supplements such as food yeast, protein supplements, meat substitutes and dried milk powders (vegetarian ones included) are used with great restraint or rarely used.

High fat levels in the blood can also lead to **neuropathy**, the distressing nervous system disorder often seen in diabetics. The symptoms range from emotional mood swings to shooting pains or burning sensations. (See Neurologic Symptoms in Chapter Eight.) Coffee and its brown beverage relatives cause **myo-inositol** to be excreted in the urine. Myo-inositol stabilizes nerves and decreases the risk of neuropathy. (See Chapter Eleven for a list of foods high in myo-inositol.)

**High salt levels** will also contribute to neuropathy. Lack of the ability to concentrate, depression, anxiety, unexplained crying, failing memory, dizziness and tingling and numbness of the feet, are all associated with elevated salt levels.

It can be seen that the **diet of the diabetic** should be 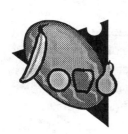 principally fruits, vegetables, especially green vegetables, and whole grains with a few nuts and seeds, as previously noted. These complex carbohydrates should be emphasized. **Garlic and onion** should be included in the diet because they have helpful properties for reducing hypoglycemic reactions and lowering elevated blood sugar in the diabetic.[60] All of these foods normalize blood sugar levels.

We no longer believe we need to restrict the intake of these complex carbohydrates-the high starch, high sugar vegetables and fruits-other than is proper to control weight or growth. If the person is not sensitive to them, they may be eaten freely. It is an individual choice based on how they are tolerated.

If anything is added to this basic diet, even oils or salt, it becomes more of a tax on the available machinery to process it, and leads to accelerated aging.

## Pre-Diabetic Syndrome

A number of separate but interrelated mechanisms appear responsible for the hypoglycemic syndrome in pre-diabetics. These include increased adrenalin, cortisol, growth hormone, rebound elevation of the sugar level and an increase in free fatty acids leading to ketonemia, which is a condition similar to starvation caused by using up body fat. Ketonemia is related to the Somogyi reaction, which is the rebound elevation of blood sugar leading to over-administration of insulin. Too much insulin can also cause severe reactions such as convulsions and in some instances, death.

Diabetics who continue to complain of hypoglycemic symptoms (See the following Symptoms of Hypoglycemia under Diabetic Emergencies.) after adjustment of the insulin dosage may be experiencing insulin-induced hypotension, which includes fainting in patients with diabetic neuropathy. Insulin-induced hypotension is not seen in the absence of neuropathy. These findings may explain patient complaints of morning attacks of confusion and weakness when blood sugar levels stand above 300. Look for postural hypotension in order to establish the diagnosis. The way to do this is with blood pressure readings as follows:

First, obtain a blood pressure reading while the person is sitting. Leave the cuff in place and have the person stand. Repeat the blood pressure reading. A fall of more than 20 points confirms a diagnosis of postural hypotension. Too rapid a change in the level of glucose, up or down, rather than the actual concentration, may be the cause of this problem.

## Diabetic Emergencies

People on insulin, with poorly controlled diabetes are always at risk for two emergency situations. The first, hypoglycemia, or very low blood sugar, can occur in both Type I and Type II diabetes, but is rare with Type II. The second emergency is

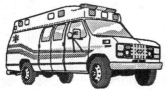

diabetic ketoacidosis. It occurs almost exclusively in Type I diabetes. You and your family must be able to recognize these two emergencies. Since immediate treatment is always critical, protect yourself and loved ones by learning to recognize early symptoms.[61]

### Symptoms of Hypoglycemia (Insulin Reaction)

Most hypoglycemic reactions come on suddenly. They can be caused by too much insulin, not enough food eaten or more exercise than usual. There will be no sugar in the urine, unless the person has not emptied the bladder in a while and sugar from a previous high blood sugar is still in the urine. Any of the following symptoms may occur: mood change, trembling, paleness, pounding heartbeat, drowsiness, inability to focus the eyes, hunger, sweating, light-headedness, confusion and disorientation, inability to concentrate and eventually, loss of consciousness. You should immediately eat a piece of fruit or some good quality food, such as whole wheat bread, cooked vegetables or some nuts, or drink a glass of fruit juice. If you are unable to swallow, take glucagon, which you should keep on hand. If you are not alert and able to take food within 25 minutes after the glucagon injection, you must be taken to the hospital. When the emergency is past, discuss your insulin or oral hypoglycemic dosage with your doctor.

### Symptoms of Ketoacidosis

Ketoacidosis develops slowly over 8-24 hours. It is caused by not having enough insulin in your body or by severe physical or emotional stress. At first there may be no symptoms. The first warning sign is a large amount of sugar--1-2%--in the urine, with a positive test for urinary acetone or ketone. You may also experience excessive thirst, excessive urination, weakness, loss of appetite, nausea, vomiting, stomach pains, rapid breathing and stupor. Later, you may feel drowsy and your breath will have a fruity odor. Certain factors increase your body's need for insulin and can cause ketoacidosis to develop quickly. These include infection, fever, vomiting, diarrhea, pneumonia and even fasting. If you become confused or unconscious, you should be taken to the hospital immediately.[62]

Reactions from the long-acting insulins (NPH, Lente, Ultralente, etc.) are different. There will often be an early change in personality; fretfulness, anger, memory loss, weakness and mild confusion. If untreated, these symptoms may progress to loss of consciousness and sometimes convulsions. Reactions during the night may cause profuse sweating and difficulty in awakening. Learn to recognize these symptoms so that they can be treated (as stated above) quickly.

### The Feet of the Diabetic

Diabetes may interfere with the circulation of blood to the legs and feet, making any minor injury slow to heal, prone to infection and dangerous. It is very important to take good care of the feet, to give them careful daily attention and to avoid injury. The person with diabetes should make it a part of the daily routine to inspect the toes for corns and calluses, and the toenails for stains or dark streaks that resemble a splinter, which may indicate the beginning of a fungus nail. If allowed to spread the fungus will ruin the nail, causing it to become thickened, deformed, dead and separated from the nail bed. It is then subject to inflammation, infection, ingrown toenail or gangrene.

If you see a **fungus nail** beginning, do not resort to the use of antifungal drugs. These drugs injure the body and when they are discontinued there is a high risk for a recurrence of the fungus. Try a home remedy instead. Scrape the dark discoloration off the nail completely with a sharp scissor or knife blade. The fungus is in the discolored area. Scrape the entire nail until it is thin. Several sessions of scraping may be required to get all the fungus off. Then apply a drop of the solution made from the following recipe twice a day:

| *fungus nail medicine* | 2 cups of vinegar |
| --- | --- |
| | $^1/_2$ oz. of myrrh |
| | $^1/_2$ oz. of calendula |

Pour all the ingredients into a glass jar with a tight lid and allow it to soak in a dark place for three weeks. Shake the jar twice daily. After three weeks, strain the solution, rinse the jar, discard the herbs and store the liquid back in the jar. You can start using the solution from the first day you mix it, even though it does not reach full potency until the three weeks end. Plain vinegar is also helpful. If you are sensitive to vinegar, use two cups of water and add two tablespoons of citric acid. You can buy citric acid at a store selling canning supplies.

Prevention is always the best strategy. The "Daily Care for the Feet of Diabetics" list in this chapter, will help you protect your toenails from fungus. One added reminder is to allow your blankets to cover your feet loosely. If blankets are laying heavily across your toes, the blood is pressed from the nail beds and this weakens the resistance of the nail to fungus. Also, keep your toenails short.

Athlete's foot can also cause serious problems for diabetics. Athlete's foot is a fungus infection of the skin, characterized by small blisters, cracks and skin peeling. It can itch, burn and swell. Shoes that are too tight, heavy non-porous socks, sweaty feet and the use of public showers and locker rooms with damp floors, all contribute to the spread of infection.

The infection can be acute or chronic. The acute form causes highly inflamed, oozing patches, little blisters, scaling and cracking, which can spread from the toes to the soles of the feet. The more chronic type begins with a crack in the skin between or under the toes and the development of loosely clinging dead skin under which is red, shiny raw tissue. It may itch, sting, burn and progress to a dry, scaly thickening of the skin covering a portion or most of the surface of the sole, and then develop into a chronic condition.

The treatment for athlete's foot must be divided into two types: one for the acute case and one for the chronic.

## *Treatment For an Acute Case of Athlete's Foot*

The toes are inflamed, cracked, weeping or oozing and may be infected, tender, red and swollen.

1. After showering, dry the feet thoroughly, especially between the toes, avoiding trauma to the toes.

2. Soak the feet for 20-30 minutes, four to six times daily in warm water no hotter then 103-104 degrees. Add one to four tablespoons of vinegar per quart of water. When the acute infection has been cleared, pure vinegar can be applied after the morning shower and allowed to air dry or dried with a blow dryer before dressing.

3. Rubbing alcohol can be applied during the day to encourage drying. Use a towel to dry between toes, because the alcohol can remain trapped between skin surfaces. After the alcohol has dried, dust feet with goldenseal powder (can stain fabrics, so use care) or cornstarch. Use clean socks after each treatment.

4. Try to avoid the use of nylon stockings. As long as the feet are acutely infected, use canvas sneakers or sandals, avoiding plastic shoes or nylon linings. Put shoes in the sun every other day and alternate pairs of shoes if possible.

5. Warm and cold alternating foot baths with no medication are also good treatments for an acute infection. Start with a warm foot bath, at about 99-102 degrees for six minutes, immediately followed by a cold foot bath using cold tap water for one minute, then back into the warm bath and follow once again with the cold. Do the warm to cold procedure three to six times. For severe cases, this treatment may be repeated every two hours. After the baths, dry feet and toes completely, using the alcohol method described above, and dust with cornstarch or goldenseal.

6. Expose the feet to sunshine for five to 20 minutes per day, depending on tolerance. This is an excellent treatment.

7. The use of Tea Tree oil has been found effective in many cases. It can be obtained from a health food store.

8. Sometimes an "id" reaction occurs. This is a painful or itching rash on the hands which appears somewhat like the rash on the feet. It is an allergic reaction to the fungus products or to overly vigorous treatments. It will subside when the inflammation of the feet calms down.

## Treatment For The Chronic, Dry, Scaly Form of Athlete's Foot

1. Apply vinegar to the feet immediately after showering each morning. Let the feet dry before dressing.

2. Since athlete's foot can make the skin more sensitive to a variety of allergenic agents, be cautious about what is applied to the feet at this stage. If you know you are sensitive to apples or apple vinegar, do not use apple vinegar as it can cause a more serious inflammation. Use dry baking soda instead. This causes the feet to be equally as alkaline as they were acid with the vinegar. Each of these discourages the growth of the fungus, although an acid condition is more effective. Use lemon juice concentrate or citric acid if you are sensitive to vinegar.

3. Keeping the feet dry with cornstarch or talc can be helpful to prevent or eradicate athlete's foot. Commercial foot remedies may contain boric acid which can be absorbed into the blood stream from irritated, open or ulcerated lesions. Boric acid irritates the kidneys. Griseofulvin is often prescribed. It is known to be toxic to unborn children and to young children. Immediate side effects include headache, mental confusion, upset digestion and serious blood disorders. Long-term effects have not been studied and have become a cause for concern.

## Herbal Remedies For Foot Soaking for Fungus Disease or Other Foot Problems

1. Goldenseal, Thyme, Garlic, Witch Hazel and Comfrey Root can be used to make water solutions. Boil one cup of water, turn flame off and add one tablespoon of an herb. Steep for 30 minutes and add to the warm foot bath. Be cautious not to let the water for the foot bath become hotter than 103-104 degrees for the diabetic. 99-102 degrees is safer for the diabetic.

2. For an alcohol-herbal preparation: Use four ounces of any herb listed above to one pint of alcohol. Let soak for two weeks and shake twice daily. At the end of two weeks, strain and store the liquid. Add one tablespoon to each quart of warm water.

3. One clove of garlic can be blended in one to two quarts of water and used as a solution to bathe the feet, or it may be applied after showering or used as an application during the day.

4. If walking is difficult, a poultice of red clover tea may be useful. Boil a cup of water, turn off the heat and add one tablespoon of tea. Let it steep for 20 minutes. Pour some of this onto a clean, cotton cloth and wrap around the affected areas of your feet. Leave on for one to six hours. Never put your shoes on if oily ointments or moist poultices are being used, because the skin of the feet will become soft and cause blisters where the shoes rub when you walk. Also, the likelihood of getting a severe inflammation is increased. (*List repeated in Chapter 12.*)

## Prevention

1. Follow the morning shower with a vigorous foot-scrubbing using a coarse, dry towel to remove the dead skin, giving particular attention to the toenails

and between the toes. This removes any extra dry skin which is the garden soil for the fungus. Rub a light coat of vinegar on the feet. Allow the feet to air dry, put on cotton socks and preferably shoes capable of evaporating sweat - sandals or loose, canvas shoes. Changing the shoes every other day to allow the moisture to fully evaporate is important.

2. Avoid public swimming pools and gymnasiums designed for walking barefoot.

## *Daily Care for The Feet of Diabetics*

The following is a list of things to do to care for your feet if you are diabetic. If you are not diabetic, these suggestions will still be helpful to you.

1. Wear stockings that are colorfast and change them at least once a day. Wash new socks before wearing them.

2. Use shoes that are pliable, but will also protect you from the trauma of bumping into furniture etc.. Learn to use a shoehorn to prevent bruising or scratching. A good brand of shoes for women is "Easy Spirit." They are expensive, but are also attractive for street wear, protective and comfortable.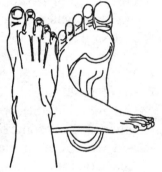

3. Wash the feet once or twice daily with a neutral soap and warm water or just plain warm water with no soap. Do not soak feet in hot water. This will raise the tissue metabolism as the temperature rises, but the blood supply of a diabetic may not be sufficient to supply the extra needs for oxygen and nutrients. Blistering can occur, which will take a very long time to heal. Dry carefully with a coarse towel, using a friction motion to keep the skin toughened. Clean the nails. Trimming should be done straight across

to discourage ingrown toenails. Above all, be gentle, but do not hesitate to rub your feet to a red glow with the towel if the skin is unbroken.

4. Shun strong antiseptics and soaps as they may cause irritations or allergic reactions. Fungicidal powders can cause the same reactions. Inspect your feet regularly. If there is any redness, pus, swelling, a sore or a crack, begin treatment right away.

5. If you use insulin, do not attempt to remove callouses or corns with chemicals or by sharp cutting with a razor blade. This is asking for considerable trouble. Have an assistant help you carefully lift the callous or corn off with your fingernail, an eyebrow tweezers or a scissors. Be extremely careful to cut only around the edges of the dead skin of the corn or callous and not into the live skin of your foot or toe. Pour a little dish detergent into a large container such as a bucket of warm water and soak your feet for 30-45 minutes. After this soaking you can usually pull a corn off with very little effort using one of the instruments listed.

6. Never wear garters or nylons with the knee-high elastic tops. Do not sit with your legs crossed, as this can strangle the circulation. Swelling of the feet invites dermatitis and infection with fungus or bacteria.

7. Sitting in a chair all day with pressure against the leg arteries, will stagnate your circulation. This encourages the development of varicose veins which can start a process that results in leg ulcers, skin rashes or pain. Give your feet as much exercise as you can, such as climbing stairs in your slippers.

8. Do not smoke. It causes the blood vessels to act as if you tied rubber bands around the ankles.

9. Do not use any kind of lubricating ointment or salve on the feet in the daytime, only at night. If you walk around with an ointment on your feet, the skin may

blister, because it is softened by the salve and it will become irritated more easily. Try to keep the feet dry always. If the feet sweat use a mild foot powder, corn starch or talcum powder.[63]

10. Never go barefoot, even around the house. Wear slippers with sturdy protective toes when shoes are not being worn. Wear sneakers or rubber sandals when at the beach or swimming.

11. Avoid sunburn of the feet.

12. Do not expose the feet to hot compresses, thermophores, heating pads, caustic solutions, or any soaking chemicals, unless your health care provider endorses it.

13. Do not use hot water bottles filled with very hot water on your feet. Use only warm water, as the nerves to the feet in diabetics often become insensitive and you may not be able to tell when the water is too hot. Bed socks may be used to keep the feet warm at night. If you must use a space heater, keep it far enough away from the bed so there is no chance of your feet touching it in your sleep. Remember that the skin of a diabetic may have greatly reduced sensation, making it impossible to recognize too much heat.

14. Gangrene of the feet and legs in diabetics should be treated by well selected exercise, not bed rest as previously recommended in standard medical treatments.[64] (See case history in Chapter Two on Diabetic Gangrene and Chapter Ten for Exercises.)

## Foot Exercises

These exercises should be done every day.

1. Lie with your legs elevated for three minutes. A good way to do this is to put a pillow on the seat of a chair, then lie on the floor, lift your legs, bend your knees and rest your legs, from your calves to your feet, on the chair.

2. Sit in the chair with your legs dangling and move your feet from the ankles, up and down and rotate

them sideways.  Do this for four minutes.
3. Cover yourself for warmth; rest five minutes.

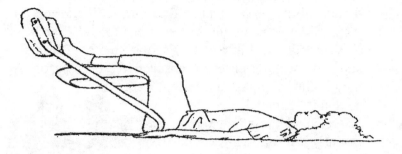

4. Stand on your feet, rock up on your toes and back on your heels ten times.  This exercise assists the circulation by promoting the health of arteries, nerves and veins.[65]

## *Health Care Habits and Diabetic Patients*

These guidelines will help you as you begin to learn new habits to improve your health.

1. Education.  For the best control, education in all facets of diabetes is desirable.  It should be given as an integral part of therapy.  The patient should become an active participant in his or her own care, and not dependent on others so far as possible.

2. Eat at set times.  Low blood sugar can cause rebound high blood sugar followed by another rebound to low blood sugar.  This occurrence is called "rebound phenomenon".  This was discussed earlier as the Somogyi effect.  It is highly desirable that both low and high sugar levels be avoided.  In general, this can be accomplished by eating foods at regular intervals, chewing thoroughly - to a cream - and eating slowly. For Type II diabetics not on long-acting insulin, it is better to fast if the meals are greatly off

schedule, rather than eat a meal several hours off the appointed hour.

3. Avoid concentrated foods. It is important to avoid very concentrated foods such as refined carbohydrates, refined proteins and refined oils. Mineral and vitamin supplements are concentrated foods also, and may precipitate high or low blood sugar. These supplements interfere in the absorptive processes, or they irritate the gastrointestinal tract so that it "dumps."

4. Exercise. Get regular exercise, especially just following a meal. Exercise is the most easily accessible treatment for most diabetic patients. Consider these facts:

   a. Muscles require energy to do their tasks.

   b. Muscles get their best energy source from glucose. This energy production requires that sugar be taken from the blood.

   c. Exercise increases muscle mass which provides more space for additional glycogen storage and helps to reduce blood glucose. Even when not exercising, the larger muscles help to stabilize blood sugar.

   d. The muscle cell becomes more insulin receptive when it is exercised, making the need for insulin decrease during exercise. Reduced production of insulin has a beneficial effect on the blood pressure and the health of the arteries. It also lessens the risk of cancer.

   e. Walking, or purposeful labor such as gardening, is usually the best exercise.

f. Exercise also improves circulation, lowers cholesterol, reduces weight and improves sleep.

g. Exercise neutralizes stress. (See section on Stress Control in Chapter Ten.)

h. Exercise combats depression and anxiety.

i. Exercise helps to control appetite. Mild exercise promotes and normalizes appetite, while heavy exercise suppresses excessive appetite.

5. Eat a high carbohydrate, low fat diet. The total vegetarian (vegan) diet, high in unrefined carbohydrates, is the most beneficial for all diabetics. A high carbohydrate, low fat diet will improve glucose tolerance and lower cholesterol levels. (See menus and recipes in Chapter 11.)

Studies have shown that blood vessel disease in diabetics is several times higher in the Western world than in underdeveloped countries. It is now recognized that the high carbohydrate diets used by Eastern physicians for controlling diabetes, rather than the high fat, high protein diets used by Western clinicians, have resulted in a decrease in blood vessel disease.

6. Daily bath. The diabetic should take a cleansing bath daily, using a mild soap or no soap at all, and rub dry with a coarse towel.[66] Women should avoid using soap on the genital area, as it tends to dryness and irritation.

7. Avoid pharmaceuticals as much as possible. Oral diabetic medications also increase cardiovascular mortality. Death rates from heart and related diseases, are twice as high among patients taking pills for their diabetes, as among those taking insulin or using diet alone. A vegetarian diet is the best ally in treating diabetes, not pharmaceuticals or insulin, ex-

cept when insulin is absolutely necessary for Type I diabetics.

## Food Budgets and Diabetes

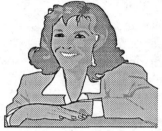 The following story explains a formula for keeping food costs down and for helping to plan menus for family members with diabetes. It was given to us by a friend who worked out the principles gradually as she searched for ways to economize, yet still create nutritious meals.

When she prepared a meal, she cooked exactly the amount of food the family needed for that meal and served the entire portion for each person on their plate. When the portion was eaten, the person was finished with their meal! The next meal could be adjusted depending on whether a family member complained of hunger or if our friend observed something or nothing left on a plate. This is called the "Russian Style" of serving. It will be easier to serve meals if each person has his or her own tray and does place setting and dishwashing for themselves. Trays that are ready and set can be stored on plastic stack shelves purchased from a department store.

Our friend shopped carefully using a complete list that she had written out earlier. She took only a specific amount of cash and never gave in to impulse buying. By watching for specials and being careful not to needlessly stock up (overstocking encourages overuse of foods), she was able to feed her family of four, in 1987, on $16.00 a week. The price of small quantities of meat was included in this figure. Vegetarians would spend even less.

She always used the smaller size packages even though these were more expensive per volume. This encouraged her to use products more sparingly. In the long run less is eaten and less money is spent. If you have a large storage area and wish to buy in quantity, the same economy can be accomplished by taking only small amounts in small containers from the storage bins. She served either a green salad or a cooked vegetable, not both, at one meal. For diabetics, a smaller number of items on the menu will improve insulin binding on cells. She cooked many meatless meals and many meals that used meat only as a flavoring agent in a dish, even though she and her family were not vegetarian. She used no junk or empty calorie foods.

By following the suggestions outlined in this chapter, you can insure yourself the best of physical health, the greatest freedom from emotional breakdowns and the slowest rate of aging possible. Plus, the entire program should save you money.

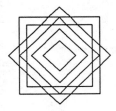

# CHAPTER SEVEN

# *Encouraging Case Histories--Diabetes*
## *and the*
# *Hypoglycemic Syndrome*

We have definite periods in our lives. If we are intemperate in any one period and become ill from our indiscretions, we may, by painstaking effort, improve our condition of health in the next period. We can then enter future periods with better health than ever experienced before. But in order to recover and preserve our health we must always follow and maintain the best health practices and routines. This calls for discipline. If you have not been very disciplined during your life, you can begin to learn discipline now. Our loving Heavenly Father has the power to help you and He is willing to give His power to the one who asks in faith.

The periods of life can be broken down into approximate lengths as follows:

| | |
|---|---|
| Newborn | |
| Early Infancy | |
| Childhood | Until 10 years of age |
| Adolescence | to 15 |
| Youth | to 25 |
| Adult | to 50 |
| Middle | to 70 |
| Old Age | to 88 |
| Advanced Old Age | 90+ |

## Encouraging Case Histories

Through the years, we have treated many patients with diabetes and hypoglycemia at Uchee Pines Institute and in our office practices. The following case histories illustrate certain complications diabetics and hypoglycemics are prone to develop. Each case is described, either by Agatha M. Thrash, M.D. or Calvin L. Thrash, M.D. The stories show the wonderful changes that take place when a patient decides to modify diet and other lifestyle practices.

### Case 1 - Diabetes Controlled by Cutting Out Fats

We received this letter from a physician acquaintance who is a recovered diabetic:

Dear Doctors Calvin and Agatha Thrash,

I know you will enjoy reading about the following experience I had.

As we are aware, it has been proven that fat reduction will reduce the need for insulin in people with diabetes mellitus. But the popular press and I think many doctors are not aware of this fact.

I stopped eating free fats for one day as a test. The next morning I had my worst hypoglycemic attack ever, as my pancreas awoke after a 10-year sleep. My theory is that just as fat globules can be seen blocking capillaries in the conjunctiva, they can also block capillaries in the pancreas. Leaving free fats out of my diet improved my pancreatic action.

The next day I took a 25-unit dose of insulin (half my usual dose), and over the course of several days I slowly decreased the dose further, watching my glucose levels in urine and blood. The levels are now normal at all times of the day, even without insulin. I don't have to bother with daily needles or fear a hypoglycemic episode, as long as I follow a diet fairly low in fat.

In medical school in 1927, we were taught that carbohydrates were the diabetic person's enemy and extra fat was needed for nourishment. The reverse is true. Think of the effect of fat on arteriosclerosis.

I consider my diabetes cured.

F. Gerard Allison, MD, FRCPC (from Vancouver, BC)

Dr. Allison believes his pancreas had been inhibited by free fats such as mayonnaise, margarine, fried foods, cooking fats, salad oils and nut butters in his diet. Removing these fats enabled him to recover from his diabetes. We are grateful for this letter which confirms our long-held belief that free fats, as well as free sugars, are the worst enemies of the diabetic.

*Case 2 - Diabetes and High Cholesterol*
A 58 year-old female school teacher arrived at the Uchee Pines Lifestyle Center as an out-patient. She had gained about 30 pounds over the past year, and in the last two or three months she had not been feeling well - decreased energy, frequent colds, and vaginal yeast infections. About ten days before, she had gone to her doctor in another city. Blood tests revealed a sugar level of 350 mg/dl. The patient was quite indignant because, "He wrote me out a prescription for some pills and said, 'You've got diabetes,' and gave me a printed out sheet from a drug company, telling me to come back in a month."

111

On examination she weighed 160 pounds at five feet, five inches, with a blood pressure of 160/90. Her fasting blood sugar was 368 and serum cholesterol was 348. I suggested a diet that was predominantly vegetarian, very low in fats and high in unrefined carbohydrates, with plenty of raw foods. I also instructed her regarding exercise and weight control.

In two weeks, she had lost six pounds and her fasting blood sugar was down to 190. In another two weeks, her fasting blood sugar had dropped to 124, and her cholesterol had dropped to 220. She continued to lose weight and to walk faithfully every morning before going to school. Within four months, she had lost 30 pounds, was feeling extremely well, and her blood sugar was normal. Her blood pressure continued to drop slowly, her cholesterol eventually reached 190 and her lowest weight was 118 pounds.

She has done quite well over the past three and a half years. Her blood sugar remains normal. She is usually very careful to avoid refined carbohydrates and free fats. Occasionally her blood pressure and cholesterol levels become slightly elevated, and her weight begins to creep upward again. This happens when she is not as careful as usual to avoid animal products and free fats.

## Case 3 - Diabetes, Hypertension and Heart Disease

A 68 year-old lawyer and former judge entered our Lifestyle Center with a diagnosis of adult onset diabetes. He was taking 65 units of NPH insulin daily. He was also on medication for hypertension and had had a heart attack several years earlier. He continued to have severe angina. He had osteoarthritis in many joints, and chronic phlebitis in both lower legs making it difficult for him to get around. He weighed 215 pounds. His blood sugar on arrival was 265 and serum cholesterol was 258. His blood pressure was 176/100, his heart was borderline enlarged and he had longstanding swelling of the lower extremities with discoloration of the lower legs and ankles.

I stopped his insulin immediately, and put him on a two-day fast. During that time, his blood pressure came down to 150/

112

90 and his blood sugar dropped to 200. He was treated with a mildly heated whirlpool to the lower extremities, massage and very mild exercise. He was given a total vegetarian, oil-free diet, high in unrefined carbohydrates. Within 3 days his blood sugar had dropped within the normal range and remained so throughout his stay except for two times when it rose to 140. His serum cholesterol came down to 186 in 3 weeks.

He returned home to continue his work of practicing law which he had given up several months before. I hear from him from time to time and after five or six years, he is continuing to do well, even though he now eats fish twice a week and occasionally drinks some milk.

### Case 4 - Diabetes and Neuropathy

In 1982, I saw a 62 year-old former accountant from Virginia, who was brought to our Lifestyle Center in a wheelchair. His health had been rapidly deteriorating during the preceding months, he was having severe pain and weakness in his lower extremities and he was nearly unable to walk. He was irritable and irascible and slept poorly. He described his pain as burning, boring and at times a tingling that did not let up. The pain was worse at night. The only pertinent history was what he had been told several years before; that he was a borderline diabetic. He was on no medication except for pain pills.

When he arrived, he was somewhat mentally clouded and had considerable difficulty concentrating and remembering. He had lost quite a bit of weight and feared that he had cancer. He had some atrophy of the muscles of the lower extremities, and on neurological examination he was found to have decreased reflexes and sensitivity to pin pricks in both legs. Laboratory data showed a fasting blood sugar of 132, and a two-hour after meal sugar of 266. His serum cholesterol was 244.

I felt he was suffering primarily from diabetic neuropathy. He was given a total vegetarian, fat-free diet that contained a number of foods high in myo-inositol (citrus fruits, cantaloupe, peanuts, beans, and whole grains-See complete list in Chapter 11.). He was also given alternating warm and cool baths to his lower extremities and passive range of motion exercises for his legs.

His blood sugar came down slowly, and after two weeks his fasting blood sugar remained in the normal range, although the after meal sugar was still elevated in the area of 180 to 200. After a week he was able to stand and walk slowly with a walker. In three weeks his blood sugars were all normal and he was able to walk over 100 yards without any assistance. His pain had virtually disappeared.

Two weeks after he returned home, he called to tell me he had gotten a CT scan that showed cancer in the abdomen, and the surgeons were planning to operate on him immediately. An exploratory operation was done, with entirely normal findings in the abdomen and no sign of cancer. Somehow the CT scan had been wrong.

He persisted with the health recovery routine and continued to improve gradually. After three months, he was essentially free from symptoms and able to go back to work.

It is frequently found that diabetic neuropathy affects the brain and central nervous system, as well as the peripheral nerves. But with changes in diet, there can be striking improvement in the emotions and mental processes, along with the disappearance of physical pain.

## Case 5 - Hypoglycemia and Fainting

Anita was 18 years old, when she suddenly fainted one morning before breakfast. She had always thought of herself as unusually healthy. She was large for her age, skilled in athletics and her friends appreciated her as the life of any party or gathering.

Because of her talents, she was asked to join many types of activities. Her drive led her to ignore her frequent colds, menstrual difficulties and frequent bouts of feeling either blue or strangely not well. The fact that she had fainted made her realize her health was not as good as she had assumed.

Anita's mother had read my material on the hypoglycemic syndrome, and recognized her daughter's condition as fitting the characteristics. She sat down with her daughter and went over the program. The whole family changed their lifestyle in order to be in harmony with the program Anita would be using. Anita's health improved steadily. Her resistance to infections improved and her periods became less troublesome. On her birthday, six months later she remarked, "I feel ten years younger than I did last year."

## Case 6 - Hypoglycemic Syndrome and Appendicitis

Jane was a high school junior when one day she began to have unrelenting abdominal pain, rising fever and no appetite. Her doctor made the diagnosis of acute appendicitis and recommended she be hospitalized immediately for surgical removal of her appendix.

The day following the surgery her father saw me in the hospital corridor just outside the pathology department. He told me of her health condition and asked why she had developed appendicitis, when none of his other four daughters had ever had such a problem.

I told him that when I had examined his daughter's appendix I had found a stone in it, typical of those who consume a high-fat, high-sugar diet. On inquiring about her health habits, it was obvious why Jane was the one who would have appendicitis.

Her father told me of Jane's great love for refined foods. She especially liked fatty foods, fried foods, chips, mayonnaise, sausage, hot dogs and all sweet foods such as ice cream and cakes. A piece of pie with a milkshake was her favorite treat. She had recently been complaining of fatigue. Jane was his tallest daughter; a bit on the plump side. None of his other daughters had insisted on the refined diet Jane loved, but enjoyed the good vegetables and fresh fruits their mother had always provided.

I explained how free sugars and free fats cause stones to form in the appendix as well as in the gall bladder. If the appendix then swells, as it might from a viral infection, the stone presses blood out of the appendix. At this point the appendix becomes inflamed and the result can be the beginning of appendicitis. I also suggested that her diet might be causing her bouts of fatigue.

Two weeks later, Jane was sent to my office by her father, for instructions on changing her lifestyle. When I went over the typical lifestyles of people with appendicitis, she recognized herself as a typical hypoglycemic. Her symptoms had been annoying, but not yet incapacitating; carious teeth, weakness, fatigue and wide mood swings. Her sisters had not experienced any of these symptoms to the severity Jane had.

Jane was highly motivated to make changes. She stopped carrying a soft drink can and began to carry a sipper bottle filled with water. She believed the water gave her a brightness she had not had before. Her mother told her it was a pleasure to cook for her now that she would eat the meals and not touch the desserts or condiments.

Jane lost weight and did not have any more cavities. By making changes so early in her life, I believe she will avoid more serious problems with hypoglycemia and even diabetes. Jane herself said, "I feel great now, better than in my entire life!"

## Case 7 - *Hypoglycemia, Behavior Problems and Heart Attack*

Walter was the 16 year-old son of a well known TV announcer in a large town. His parents brought him to see me because of his unpleasant attitude at home and his general poor health.

His appearance was one of strength and vitality. He was nearly six feet tall and husky, but with a very guarded, almost hostile expression on his face.

For over an hour I tried to explain to Walter why he had health problems and a negative attitude towards life. Several times during this interview, I was interrupted by his parents who argued and pleaded with him to listen. He refused to listen to them or to me, and finally said to his parents, "Let's go, I'm not going to do anything different."

Walter's parents continued to have trouble with him and he moved out of their home at age 18. He was unable to communicate with his parents in a positive manner for 15 years. His life was troubled and turbulent.

He married young, divorced a year later and was frequently sick with allergies. His weight rose to 220 pounds from his habit of eating rich foods in restaurants. When he was 30 years old, he suddenly suffered a heart attack. At that point he came to see me again.

After he had several tests, it was found that his cholesterol was 285, triglycerides were 350, and his fasting blood sugar was 116mg%. His cardiologist had told him he had to lose weight or he would die with his next heart attack.

Walter had a serious struggle with the discipline required to begin and maintain a good health recovery program. His mother offered to begin the program with him, adding that she would prepare his meals and invited him to eat at his parent's home. I went over the program with her. She enthusiastically changed her menus, as both she and her husband also wanted to lose weight.

Ten years later, Walter's weight was 50 pounds less than at the time of his heart attack. His cholesterol was 170, triglycerides were 84 and his blood sugar was 88. He married a young lady who worked at a health spa. She was pleased to provide a healthful diet for them both. Life is improving for Walter. Some of us, like Walter, have to learn life's lessons the hard way.

### Case 8 - Hypoglycemia and Behavior Problems

It was spring when I met 13 year-old Valerie. During my interview with Valerie and her mother, she turned her back on me. She showed no evidence of even recognizing my presence, except by an occasional exclamation of "That's weird," or "Huh."

Her mother had not been able to give direction and discipline to her daughter during Valerie's first 13 years of life. I had little hope that she would be able to do these things now. Valerie was an unfortunate victim of her home environment and she suffered uncontrollable mood swings. She did not do well at school, had poor grades and no friends. In spite of my conflicting feelings, I wrote out three pages of health program instructions, making certain her mother understood them all.

Because of prior scheduling and summer vacation, I was not able to see Valerie again until one week after school started. I was dreading the encounter and hoped she would not come back for her appointment if she had made no changes. But on the afternoon of our appointment, as I gazed out of my office window, I saw Valerie and her mother in the parking lot.

Valerie walked immediately into my office without stopping at the front desk. She threw a paper on my desk which had a test score of 100 at the top. I looked up at her to see a great big smile. "That is the first one of those I have ever made," she said. Valerie was a transformed 14 year-old.

I was delighted with the story her mother told me. "Valerie and I sat down to have the first real heart-to-heart talk we ever had," she began, "after we left your office three months ago. I asked her if she was happy with her life and wanted to continue fighting with everybody for as long as she lived, or if she would like to change. I told her she was now at a crossroads and could make a change if she wanted to. To my surprise, she said she wanted to change. At first I was stunned and could not say anything. But when I found my voice I took out your instructions and told her they all seemed reasonable to me, and we could give them a try. She agreed."

Unlike Walter (Case #7), Valerie made changes in her lifestyle early enough to avoid crippling disease and emotional turmoil.

The last time I saw Valerie, she was 22 years-old and had come to see me for her premarital workup. I am certain she would never have settled down to a satisfying lifestyle without becoming more regular in her daily habits and without making changes in diet and exercise. She had discovered she was highly sensitive to her favorite drinks and sweet foods: coffee, tea, colas, chocolate and sugar. Her behavior became uncontrollable a few minutes after drinking or eating any of these. She would cry without cause and sometimes have wide mood swings; wildly happy and laughing loudly or hostile and disagreeable. The book *Sugar Blues*, by William Duffy, which relates in detail certain behaviors attributable to sugar consumption, could have been written about Valerie.

## Case 9 - Hypoglycemia Uncontrolled with Eight Daily Feedings

A patient from Canada came to our Lifestyle Center. He was overweight, nervous, jittery and generally did not feel well. He had been diagnosed as hypoglycemic and two years earlier his doctor had put him on six to eight feedings per day. His last meal was scheduled for 11p.m. each evening.

He was very frustrated with this routine and told me, "I have to get up early in the morning for work, and then I have to stay up until 11 o'clock at night so I can eat that last meal." I asked him, "How would you like to try a two-meal a day schedule?" And he replied, "Oh, I would die. I'm sure I would die." I answered, "Well, let's check it out."

I put him on two regular meals per day. The food was vegetarian, composed of unrefined carbohydrates with plenty of fiber for slow absorption. After five days he said, "I feel better than I have in years! I can't believe it! Why didn't the other doctors do this? I've been staying up for the past two and a half years until 11 o'clock to have my last feeding and all I had to do was cut down the amount of food I was eating and change my eating habits."

He experienced large improvements in his health. Since he also had a high stress level due to his work situation, I felt he would make advances with his health only with major changes in his work. I suggested that he needed to consider either changing the way he worked or look into the possibility of another career. I never suggest this without having a great deal of concern and respect for a patient, as we are all aware of the difficulties involved in making a vocational change. But health is the most treasured earthly possession and it is more valuable than a specific job.

\* \* \* \* \* \* \* \* \* \* \* \* \* \* \* \* \* \*

These cases show the reversals in the course of diseases and the striking improvements in health which can be made with changes in diet and exercise habits. These changes are simple ones to make, but changing the habits of a lifetime is never easy. Determination to achieve better health and many prayers to our loving Father, will help you begin and maintain the Health Recovery Program and experience your own healing.

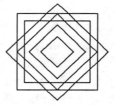

# CHAPTER EIGHT

# *The Hypoglycemic Syndrome*

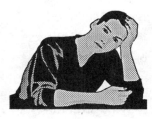 A person does not suddenly change from being normal to being a Type II diabetic. He or she often goes through a phase of the hypoglycemic syndrome with its general symptoms of fatigue and headache, its nervous system symptoms of depression and mental inefficiency and various digestive system problems.

The hypoglycemic syndrome has actually been misnamed. An accurate definition of the term "hypoglycemia" indicates that it is a disorder of carbohydrate metabolism only. The truth is that there is not a single known nutrient uninvolved in this syndrome, including vitamins, minerals, proteins, fats and even water. Protein toxicity or fat overload can have as many health consequences as sugar sensitivity.

## *Four Types*

1. *Alimentary* - This type is caused by rapid digestion and assimilation of nutrients and rapid clearing of sugar from the blood due to an overactive thyroid, excessive exercise, high stress or an unusually active metabolism. The stomach has lost its ability to recognize signals that control the rate at which food is

emptied and it expels too much food, too soon. Normally, within a few seconds after food reaches the small intestine, a virtual explosion occurs, which we call digestion. Large amounts of the tiny exploded fragments of food then pour into the blood stream.

2. *Reactive* - This type is caused by several factors: an inability of the stomach to hold food long enough for the essential processes of good digestion to occur. There may also be a failure on the part of the stomach to secrete appropriate digestive substances. The small bowel may be incapable of functioning properly and may fail to regulate the production of chemicals for the most optimum digestion. Some of these digestive enzymes can cause insulin to be secreted. And especially overeating, taking large mouthfuls, not chewing thoroughly and eating in a rush may cause this type of hypoglycemia.

Even a diet of unrefined foods can cause this type of syndrome. The pancreas and liver may be structurally normal, but the pancreas may be overly sensitive and produce too much insulin or too little glucagon. When food is eaten which has a relatively large amount of refined carbohydrates, like sugar and white flour products, the blood sugar will go up too high too rapidly. Many endocrine organs react to this rise in blood sugar and some react quite quickly. The pancreas of the sensitive person overreacts by putting out too much insulin. The blood sugar then drops quickly below the normal levels, causing symptoms. There is also a significant increase in stress hormone production.

If the person is a hypersensitive hypoglycemic, and the auxiliary digestive organs are either not ready or not capable of handling the amount of food being fed them, much havoc will occur in the nervous, circulatory, hormone and hepatic systems. For this reason, the traffic of food through the stomach has to be carefully regulated. The controlling signals may be lost due to poor health habits-eating too much or too frequently, too many foods at one meal, eating refined foods, etc.

3. *Flat tolerance curve* - This kind shows up on the glucose tolerance test as a pattern which does not follow the usual steep curve upward and then downward of a normal test. (See Chapter Two for a normal curve.) The flat curve hypoglycemic may represent a missed high blood sugar phase which occurred earlier than 30 minutes. This indicates that the blood was not tested at the correct time and so did not reveal the high level. The high level may have occurred at 15 minutes and then quickly fell before the 30 minute blood sample was withdrawn from the vein. The flat curve may also be due to poor movement and stagnation in the stomach or low thyroid function.

4. *Insulinoma (tumor of the pancreas)* - This type of tumor grows in the pancreas and produces insulin independent of the body's control. It may also give a flat curve with the glucose tolerance test.

## *Insulin and Protein Metabolism*

How insulin influences protein metabolism is not as widely appreciated as its effect on glucose and fats. It has been demonstrated that insulin causes a fall in amino acids, the building blocks of proteins, in the blood. Speculation exists as to whether the primary action of insulin is in the liver, which is the major site for deamination (the beginning step in the breakdown of proteins and amino acids), or in muscle where the bulk of the body protein reserves lie.

The role of insulin, in suppressing the release of amino acids by muscle tissue, was shown by directly introducing insulin into the forearm muscle of a man who was fasting. During a fast, insulin levels fall in the blood and amino acids flow from the muscle to the liver for deamination. They are then either oxidized for energy or converted to glucose or fat for immediate energy storage. Fasting therefore helps get rid of excess protein. It has only recently been understood that excess protein increases the risks of kidney disease, liver disease, cancer and heart attack.

Glucagon and insulin together, control amino acid metabolism. The effects of glucagon are opposite to those of insulin. Glucagon stimulates gluconeogenesis (conversion of stored glycogen to glucose), whereas insulin inhibits this process. The primary action of glucagon appears to take place in the liver.

Glucagon is facilitative rather than regulatory. It is secreted by the pancreas in response to incoming amino acids when there is a need for glucose production. Glucagon then stimulates conversion of the amino acids to glucose. The effect of insulin on this process can be enhanced by exercise. Insulin makes sure the conversion process is held in proper balance. The mechanisms for this are intricate and highly effective when they work correctly. Many factors can upset a portion of the mechanism, such as eating too much or between meals, stress, illness, alcohol, caffeinated beverages and pharmaceuticals, including over-the-counter drugs.

Hypoglycemia may be associated with endocrine disorders other than pancreatic. Adrenalin production, the adrenal cortical hormones, the thyroid and other organs may also be affected.

## A Nation of Hypoglycemics

The Bible says in Ezekiel 16:49 : "Behold, this was the iniquity of thy sister Sodom, pride, fullness of bread, and abundance of idleness...neither did she strengthen the hand of the poor and needy."

Because of our affluence, Americans can afford to eat expensive and exotic foods in any desired quantity, at any time of day or night and at any season of the year. Distorted habits of food consumption such as eating too much at irregular hours and taking the wrong kinds of food, become the result of this availability of food. Thirty million Americans are overweight;

some are grossly obese. On one hand we have a preoccupation with food, and on the other hand we are obsessed with becoming and staying slim.

"Fullness of bread and abundance of idleness," have made us a nation of hypoglycemics. Even those who do not suffer from overweight often have the hypoglycemic syndrome of mental confusion, emotional upsets, fatigue, allergies, gastrointestinal disorders, heart symptoms and often a complete breakdown in life. This breakdown can be emotional, mental, social or physical.

Many of these individuals are very often considered neurotic by their physicians, because there seem to be no physical reasons for their problems. They appear "strong and healthy" and yet they have reached a point of physical distress that compels them to seek medical aid. When the doctor says the illness is "all in their heads," these patients may be ready to accept this mysterious evaluation as an ex- 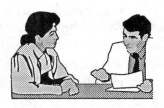 planation for their emotional and mental symptoms. Their spouses, or others close to them, may also have noted a change in their personalities.

Next may begin a futile round of visits to physicians and psychiatrists and possibly even operations or hospitalizations for testing or diagnostic procedures. But the sometimes minor alterations in the blood chemistries of glucose, cholesterol, triglycerides, uric acid and hemoglobin, which are inconsistent with the patient's age, are not recognized as representing a disabling symptom-complex (hypoglycemic syndrome). Alterations of this magnitude are seen in many test results of Americans who are not yet suffering from any kind of complaint, so physicians tend to think these changes are unimportant. Yet, there are many disorders that must be judged by a combination of several diagnostic factors, a proper history, the presence or absence of physical findings and the appropriate laboratory profile. The hypoglycemic syndrome is one of these disorders.

### Why Doctors Don't Recognize This Pattern

We believe the answer to that question lies in several factors. Some of these are outlined as follows:

1. Hypoglycemia is a physiological term referring to a transient state of the biochemistry of the blood that may or may not be associated with symptoms. All doctors have been taught this fact and tend to dismiss the laboratory results as being merely transitory.

2. There is a widespread failure to recognize that this is a far-reaching lifestyle disorder experienced by millions of people throughout the world. Because it is so extensive it is usually regarded as normal.

3. It is not normal to feel bad. Since so many people do feel bad, doctors generally tend to believe nothing should be done for this class of sufferers.

4. There is a failure on the part of doctors to recognize that the chemistry of the blood is associated with wide mood swings and even in alterations in the brain's ability to process information. Not everyone who complains of vague symptoms is a hypochondriac, in fact, most people probably have a physical or chemical disorder of some kind.

5. Evolution of our knowledge about the functions of insulin and insulin receptors is only now allowing us to clearly focus on explanations and solutions. Very few physicians, even those working in the field of metabolic disorders, are acquainted with the importance of lifestyle factors, diet and exercise in altering cellular receptors for insulin.

In no phase of the practice of medicine does an accurate diagnosis pay such large dividends in the salvage of a person's productivity as here, since the treatment routine is often spectacularly successful. We have used the "Health Recovery Routine" with a large number of patients and have seen many satisfactory results. It is simple, but requires rigid attention to detail, especially at first, as the biochemical processes that we expect to be restored are described by metabolism experts as "permanently changed." But these "permanent changes" can be reversed with persistent effort. Just as the liver and its associated organs "learned" to process foods incorrectly, they can also "learn" to process foods more normally. Body cells can "learn" to alter their way of handling nutrients. With steady retraining, the liver and other organs can be "taught" to change their metabolism back to a healthful mode.

One must not be easily discouraged in treating the hypoglycemic syndrome. While many symptoms may clear overnight, some annoying symptoms may persist almost unabated for a year or more. Eventually health will be recognized as being better.

We had one patient whose ears remained "stopped up" for over a year after beginning a good health program. Then suddenly, the blockage began to clear. What had finally caused this clearing was the restoration of good hydration. Chronic dehydration is a very common component of this syndrome. Ringing in the ears, heart palpitations, and a sense of weakness are often difficult to conquer. Faithful adherence to every detail of the program usually brings complete or nearly complete recovery.

## Do You Have The Hypoglycemic Syndrome?

Read this section and ask yourself the following questions to determine if you may be having symptoms of the hypoglycemic syndrome.

1. Review the typical symptoms, signs, and laboratory findings given in the diabetes section of this book. Have you experienced any of these signs and symptoms? Have your test results been confusing or borderline, even if they seemed insignificant to your physician?

2. What is your history of surgical procedures? Many people start off the progression of the hypoglycemic syndrome with a series of surgical procedures. The

same factors which caused symptoms resulting in an operation are also capable of causing chronic illness. Fatty or sugary junk foods promote both appendectomies and tonsillectomies, and are also causative in the development of the hypoglycemic syndrome.

3. How do you handle food biochemically? Do you ever have sugar in the urine? Do your fasting blood sugar and your two-hour after meal blood sugar readings fall within the ideal range of 70-85mg.%? No sugar should be spilled in the urine by normal kidneys in people who do not have diabetes. In a person with hypoglycemia who has normal kidneys, sugar will not show up in the urine. The ideal range for all blood sugar values, except the 30 minute and one hour readings, should be between 70 and 85. Any reading above or below this ideal may mean trouble ahead.

4. This disease does not come on without warning. There are signals all along the way, from birthweight over eight pounds, physical growth that is too rapid in infancy and childhood, on through the dental caries and teenage depressions or rebellions. Finally the blood chemistry begins to show a higher or lower than ideal blood sugar, and higher than ideal blood lipids. Ideal cholesterol is 100 plus your age, and ideal triglycerides are 100 or below, preferably nearly the same as your age. (See number ten in the Appendix for a list of blood test values.)

## *Hope For You*

The first step in the recovery from hypoglycemia is to encourage a spirit of hopefulness in yourself. Remember that your condition can be controlled and there are things you can do to help yourself.

You must train your appetite to relish our *classical* American diet with a high percentage of fruits, whole grains, nuts and vegetables, and a low percentage of animal products and white, refined foods. This diet built up a hardy breed of intelligent, hardworking citizens and made America a great world power energized by these strong, healthy people. This new approach is based on knowledge gained from our ancestors and from studies of contemporary native peoples, and has brought success in difficult to handle hypoglycemic cases.

## *Weight Control Essential*

1. Control the total calorie intake. Emphasize unrefined carbohydrates and reduce fat content.
2. Maintain ideal body weight at 5-10% below the American average. (See Chapter Ten for "Rule of Thumb for Average Weight.")
3. Maintain a regular meal schedule. This promotes better digestion. When a regular exercise program is also begun, digestion is further improved.
4. There is no need to restrict unrefined carbohydrates. Hypoglycemics are able to handle carbohydrates better than either fats or proteins. When unrefined carbohydrates are restricted, fats and proteins have been over-used to make up sufficient calories for weight maintenance.
5. One way to calculate your approximate nutrient needs is as follows: multiply your ideal body weight in pounds by 10 to get the daily recommended total calorie count. Divide the total number of calories by 5-7 to get the grams of carbohydrate. Again divide the total number of calories by 25-30 to get the grams of protein. Then divide the protein grams by 9 to get the grams of fat.

Example: A five foot tall woman, who weighs 100 pounds, should eat approximately 1000 calories per day. She should have about 200 grams of carbohydrate, 40 grams of protein and four and one-half grams of fat. One tablespoonful is approximately 12-15 grams depending on the density of food or fluid.

Although hypoglycemia has presented difficult problems in the past due to misdiagnosis or improper treatment, with the current advances in our understanding of this disorder, we have obtained positive results from a very simple and workable program. This program is described in Chapter Nine under "Health Recovery Program."

## Incidence of Hypoglycemia

There appears to be twice as many cases of hypoglycemia diagnosed as cases of diabetes. Thirty million hypoglycemic cases have been diagnosed in the United States alone. This condition is found more often in women than in men and commonly occurs between the ages of 20-30 years. Diagnosis is positive when a blood sugar reading below 60 is established, if typical symptoms are also present and no other cause can be identified. It is to be highly suspected with a reading from 65-60 and moderately suspected between 69 to 65.

## Evolution of Typical Signs and Symptoms

1. During pregnancy, the mother has food cravings
2. Birth weight over eight pounds
3. Sugar in formula-was not breast fed
4. Childhood evolution of changes:
   A. Frequent cavities in the teeth
   B. GI symptoms-may be partly due to glucagon
      a. Appendicitis
      b. Hemorrhoids
      c. Constipation
      d. Other bowel problems
      e. Peptic ulcers
   C. Virus diseases-cold hands and feet, tonsillitis
   D. Diet leads to rapid maturity
      a. Snacking
      b. Large suppers
      c. High calorie, high protein and high fat diet
      d. Milk and high intake of dairy products
         (leucine leads to increased insulin pro-

duction with increased appetite and decreased blood sugar). Calcium increases appetite
      e. Chromium deficiency
      f. Caffeine drinks
   E. Blood alterations
      a. Increased cholesterol
      b. Uric acid elevated
      c. EEG shows poor glucose utilization
      d. Excess glucagon leads to increased growth hormone
      e. Excess insulin leads to increased rate of atherosclerosis, obesity, hypertension, cancer and diabetes
      f. Irregularity in lifestyle

      g. Stress
            •TV
            •Caffeine drinks
            •Tense lifestyle
   F. Muscle biopsy shows increased blood vessel wall thickness which inhibits blood flow
   G. Insulin receptors on cells may be decreased and pancreatic pulses of insulin may be irregular

The evolution of these signs and symptoms are essentially the same as those leading to diabetes. The hypoglycemic syndrome is usually the forerunner of diabetes and can cause troublesome symptoms by itself and complicate the problems of the diabetic. A glucose tolerance test must be performed to determine if these signs are suggestive of hypoglycemia or diabetes. A low fasting blood sugar reading reveals hypoglycemia, while a high reading points to diabetes. A diabetic may have hypoglycemic reactions when experiencing the rebound effect - the fast rise in blood sugar followed by a fast drop - brought on by too much insulin.

## Psychiatric, Neurologic and Physical Symptoms

Hypoglycemia is also responsible for many of the emotional disturbances seen today in our society. It is a frequent source of disability causing many hospital beds to be filled with those suffering the negative symptoms brought on by this disorder.

As we discussed in Chapters Two and Seven, there is impaired brain metabolism with hypoglycemia, due to an inadequate glucose supply to the brain. This leads to sympathetic nervous system reactions. These reactions are often a prominent feature of the hypoglycemic syndrome. The mental changes from this SNS activity include emotional instability, confusion and occasionally coma or convulsions. When the blood sugar falls sharply, adrenalin is discharged into the blood with its characteristic train of symptoms such as palpitations, tremor, profuse sweating, pallor, panic attacks and headache.

## Major Psychological Symptoms in 300 Cases of Hypoglycemic Syndrome

This list identifies the predominant mental changes that can occur with a chronic hypoglycemic condition. The emotional changes can be the most noticeable ones.

| | |
|---|---|
| Anger | Insomnia |
| Anxiety | Irritability |
| Bizarre thoughts | Lack of concentration |
| Compulsions | Marriage problems |
| Conscientious, driving personality | Negativism |
| | Ornery streak |
| Crying spells | Phobias |
| Depression | Previous psychosis |
| Forgetfulness or confusion | Problem children |
| Frustration | Restlessness |
| Inability to complete small tasks without repeated rechecking | Suicide threats |
| | Tense personality |

## Major Neurologic Symptoms

Just as troublesome as the psychological symptoms and possibly just as obvious may be symptoms indicating nerve involvement.

| | |
|---|---|
| Abdominal spasms | Muscular twitching, cramps, |
| Bloating and gas | pains or backache |
| Blurred vision | Nervousness |
| Body symptoms anywhere | Numbness |
| Chronic indigestion | Palpitations |
| Cold hands or feet | Scalp symptoms-sensation |
| Convulsions | of water dripping, ants |
| Dizziness and nausea | crawling or a band |
| Excessive hunger | around the head |
| Exhaustion or fatigue | Staggering |
| Exhaustion or fatigue | Sweating |
| Fainting or blackouts | |
| Fast heart rate | Thick, high-pitched voice |
| Headaches | Tinnitus (ringing in ears) |
| Heart attacks | Tremors |
| Joint pains | Weakness |
| Lack of appetite | |

## Physical Signs and Symptoms Suggesting A Need For A Corrective Program

There are also certain obvious physical signs of hypoglycemia. Some of these signs may precede the psychological signs by many years.

| | |
|---|---|
| Acne | More than five dental |
| Allergies | fillings by age 20 |
| Arthritis | More than five missing |
| | teeth by age 30 |
| Cataracts | |
| Diabetes | Obesity |
| Diarrhea | Parkinsonism |
| Erythrocytosis-too many | Rapid growth in early |
| red blood cells | childhood |

Hypothyroidism
Increased blood clotting
Involuntary jumping or
    jerking
Low resistance to disease
    with frequent colds,
    sore throats, boils,
    skin and nail problems

Slow healing
Tonsillectomy
Resting heart rate over 80

## Internal Changes

In hypoglycemia, many internal changes are happening that are not as easily seen as the symptoms described in the lists e alterations in body chemistry and organ function lead to a slowing down or speeding up of the inner workings of the body and result in other disease processes. The stomach dumps food too rapidly, the colon becomes sluggish and polyps and diverticula may appear. The pancreas develops a weakness which involves both enzyme and hormone production, and the Islets of Langerhans may be damaged. The liver can no longer properly handle its role in controlling the blood sugar level.

With overuse of sugar the cells of the body, especially those in the nervous system, become injured. In severe hypoglycemic cases some symptoms are generated due to rapid falls in sugar levels and cause the inward sensations of trembling, sweating, fast heartbeat, weakness and hunger. Slower falls in sugar cause headache, coma, convulsions, transient "strokes," aberrant behavior and other signs of impaired brain function, such as the symptoms shown in the psychiatric and neurologic lists.

## Interpretation of Glucose Tolerance Test

1. The ideal fasting range is narrow: 70-85mg%. At the two hour level the blood sugar should again reach the fasting ideal or drop a few points down.
2. Some patients have symptoms with a blood sugar level between 60 and 70. Most people will have symptoms of hypoglycemia when the blood sugar falls below 60.

3. We can make the diagnosis of hypoglycemia if either of the following is found:
    a. A drop of 10-20mg below the fasting level in the glucose tolerance test.
    b. A drop of more than 50mg in one-half hour.
4. If the rate of fall in the 90 minute period immediately preceding the low exceeds one milligram per minute; or if any part of the glucose tolerance test, after the first hour, falls at a rate of one milligram per minute or more, you should suspect the diagnosis of hypoglycemic syndrome.
5. From the highest peak to the lowest valley the blood sugar reading should not be more than 100, and even 90 is suspicious.

Normal, Diabetic and Hypoglycemic Curves

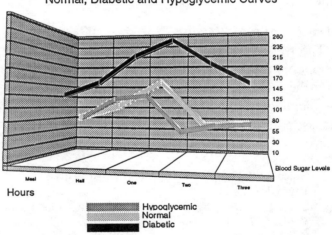

Hypoglycemia which occurs while you are fasting is more serious and difficult to treat than reactive hypoglycemia, which occurs after you have eaten. It can sometimes indicate a tumor or liver disease. Islet cell tumors of the pancreas cause blood sugar levels of 50 or less in a person who has been fasting for 48 hours or more.

Functional hypoglycemia usually gives a normal or only slightly low reading while fasting, but falls to uncomfortable levels at four to seven hours after a meal. Fasting for two or three days would cause little discomfort, but meals may be followed by much unpleasantness.

## Three Different Types of Blood Sugar Curves in Hypoglycemia

You may determine the type of hypoglycemic syndrome you have by comparing your lab tests with these figures.

|  | Flat curve | Reactive | Diabetic with Hypoglycemic Phase |
|---|---|---|---|
| Fasting | 68 mg% | 68 mg% | 88 mg% |
| 30 min. | 90 | 135-170 | 135 |
| 1 hour | 90 | 110 | 190 |
| 2 hours | 75 | 79 | 150 |
| 3 hours | 78 | 40 | 69 |
| 4 hours | 74 | 68 | 64 |
| 5 hours | 62 | 75 | 72 |

## Ideal Laboratory Reports

The hypoglycemic will be out of the ideal range in the laboratory reports given below. The ideal values are different from the average American values. Approximately 50% of the people diagnosed within the average values will die of heart disease and 40% will develop cancer. We can see these are not "normal," but only average American.

Glucose 70-85
Thyroid  4-12
Cholesterol 100 + age
Triglycerides 100 or below
Uric acid  2-5

BUN 4-15
Sodium 134-140
WBC  3000 to 5000
Hemoglobin below 5000ft.
elevation:
Female  10.5-12.5
Male    12.0-14.75

## Factors Which Control Blood Sugar

There are other body processes to take into consideration when we think about factors which govern the regulation of blood sugar. The kidneys take up large amounts of insulin which enables them to transport glucose into the urine. The ovaries and testes influence the production of insulin and glucagon. Alimentary hyperglycemia is the condition of a high thyroid function which causes a rapid uptake of sugar from the bowel. It may also occur from unknown causes. Activities in the brain which are processed by the hypothalamus affect sugar levels. Such activities can be thoughts, emotions, physical or chemical stress, all of which are aggravated by incorrect eating.

Besides improving our eating habits, one thing we can all do to help the body regulate blood sugar accurately is to begin and conscientiously maintain a program of exercise.

## Health Recovery Program

We have seen in the preceding chapters how eating habits have been studied in relation to diabetes. These studies revealed the major role which diet plays in resolving the hypoglycemic syndrome and diabetes. If you decide to embark upon the Health Recovery Program, careful attention to all dietary details is required to insure success.

80% of overweight adults develop diabetes, with significant numbers of them going through a period of the hypoglycemic syndrome on the way to fullblown diabetes. Probably 95% or more of these diabetics could be cured simply by following the Health Recovery Program.

The program must be followed for a full year before making any decisions on its effectiveness. Symptoms may clear up rapidly, or very slowly during this period. If symptoms take longer than a year to diminish there is a strong probability of food sensitivities. An elimination and challenge diet should be followed to determine those foods causing the problem. (See Elimination and Challenge diet in Chapter Eleven) Those who have a flat glucose tolerance curve can expect to be more resistant to treatment.

Use the Health Recovery Program in Chapter Nine for treating hypoglycemia. When any symptoms persist, in spite of attempts at dietary treatment, most likely the diet and other health recovery recommendations have not been followed strictly enough. Recommendations will also be discussed in Chapter Nine.

# Diet, Exercise and the Health Recovery Program

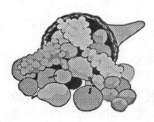 Now come the instructions on how to make a big lifestyle change. If you truly desire to regain your health, these measures will seem like simple steps to take in order to reach your aspirations. Those who are chosen to become astronauts must go through a much more rigorous training. Even though their goals are the moon and the planets, they have far less to gain than you do.

Plan to stick to the program, without deviation, for twelve months. To acquire tastes for new recipes and routines takes time. That which at first may seem strange to your palate will become quite tasty in a short period of time. Don't make snap judgments or hasty statements. Give yourself time, have patience and be open-minded about your own recovery rate. Time is in your favor!

For menu suggestions see the menu planner and recipes in Chapter Eleven, and the *Eat For Strength*, Oil-Free cookbook.[67] We recommend that you follow the oil-free diet, at least for the first year.

The following are our recommendations for the treatment of diabetes and hypoglycemia. These recommendations have proven successful for patients we have worked with in the Lifestyle Center at Uchee Pines Institute.

## Foods Allowed

### Meats

A vegetarian diet promotes healing and slows down aging better than any other type of diet. However, if meat and eggs are eaten, they should be overcooked to try to kill germs, and trimmed and blotted to remove as much fat as possible. Limit their use in accordance with the recommendations of the American Heart Association to two to five times a week. Objectionable meats such as pork, ham, bacon, sausage, shellfish of all kinds, hot dogs, hamburger, canned meat spreads, pressed meats and canned composite meats such as Spam, should all be permanently eliminated. There are recipes in *Eat For Strength* which are very acceptable meat substitutes.

### Cheese

There are cheeses, butters and sauces made from nuts, potatoes, carrots, tomatoes, onions and other vegetables and seasonings, that provide delightful creams, spreads and dips for vegetables, pastas and breads. Simple and inexpensive dishes can be made with appropriate recipes. (See *Eat For Strength*, Oil-Free edition.)[68] Dairy cheese cannot be made healthful by any kind of kitchen maneuver and must be eliminated.

### High Protein Meat Substitutes

These products are best used as a temporary measure while making the change to the vegetarian diet. They are more  healthful than meats, but not as good for you as the unconcentrated, unrefined foods from which these products were made. The meat substitutes are generally manufactured from soybeans and grains. It should be emphasized that all concentrated foods should be used sparingly and mainly as seasonings.

## Breads

Use only whole grains. Two or three different grains may be mixed for a single bread. Bread should be thoroughly cooked, and chewed well.

## Cereals

Use only whole grains. Commercial cream of wheat is not a whole grain. If you like cream of wheat, substitute bulgur wheat or farina or use the recipe in *Eat For Strength,* [69] using whole kernel wheat to make cream of wheat. You may also make cream of rice, cream of corn or cream of any whole grain. Some other easily prepared whole grain cereals are oatmeal, steel-cut oats, granola (without oil or honey), wheat cereals, buckwheat, barley, millet, brown rice, grits and whole wheat macaroni. Soy spaghetti is also acceptable.

## Vegetables

Vegetables may be used in liberal quantities. The very starchy vegetables such as Irish potatoes, corn, sweet potatoes, split peas and dried beans, may be used as main dishes instead of meat, milk, eggs and cheese. Cracked or whole kernel grains such as rice, millet, wheat, rye, barley and corn make excellent main dishes. Starchy pastas such as spaghetti and macaroni may also be eaten as long as the whole grain pasta is used. Eating these carbohydrate-rich foods is contrary the high protein, high fat diets once was recommended for this disorder. A single serving when used as a main dish should contain 250 to 300 calories. Those who are very active such as young men and pregnant or lactating mothers, may need seconds.

## Milk Products

Dairy milk products are not recommended. Milk sensitivity is the most common form of food sensitivity in the United States. Many symptoms that have obscure or unknown causes have their origin in the use of milk. There is invariably a gastrointestinal problem in persons with the hypoglycemic syndrome. Leaving milk out of the diet will benefit some of these individuals in an almost unbelievable way.

## Milk Substitutes

Recommended are nut milks, soy milks without sweeteners homemade from soybeans or flours (most commercial soy milks are heavily sweetened), cheeses made from nuts, flours or vegetables and sour and sweet creams made from special recipes. These milks may be used sparingly in cooking and in limited quantities with meals.

## Nuts and Seeds

Use all kinds sparingly, as well as their butters (peanut butter, almond butter, sesame butter, etc.). Wash shelled raw nuts in cool water and sterilize them in the oven at 225 until dry. Raw nuts, sunflower, pumpkin, sesame and other seeds may feel gummy while drying. Stirring occasionally hastens drying. Use nuts raw, or lightly roasted.

## Coffee and Tea Substitutes

All beverage herb teas are acceptable: Lemon Grass, Gossip, Red Zinger, Lemon Mint and similar blends. Postum, Caphag, Pero and other coffee substitutes are also acceptable. Some of these types of beverages have unacceptable sweeteners in them such as molasses, malt, maltose, maltodextrin or sugar beet residues. Check labels carefully. Remember that tea and coffee substitutes should be light drinks, not hearty, rich and nourishing. The only nourishing ingredient is water. All the rest is coloring, flavoring or sweetening. Teas may be sweetened with stevia powder (an herb).

## Artificial Sweeteners

It is best to learn to eat foods in their natural, unsweetened state as much as possible. One should cultivate the habit of leaving sweeteners out of food. The long-term safety of artificial sweeteners has not been established.

## Fruits

All fresh fruits and all fruits canned in water-pack or natural juices may be used, unless you know you have a sensitivity to them. Bear in mind that fruit juices should be classed as refined foods because they have had the fiber removed. Some highly sensitive individuals may need to avoid all fruits for one to three months. In this case, two vegetable meals should be eaten.

## Miscellaneous

Green or black olives (not stuffed) and avocado are tasty and nutritious. Coconut, fresh or unsweetened and grated, may be used quite safely by vegan vegetarians, as it will not usually elevate blood cholesterol in those not eating animal 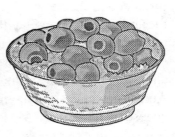 protein. There may be a temporary blood cholesterol elevation when one makes the transition from an animal product diet to a vegan diet. This happens because cholesterol is being expelled from the tissues into the blood as it is being transported out of the body.

## Foods and Drugs to Avoid

### Sugars

White, brown and raw sugar, fructose, honey (for diabetes and hypoglycemics no type of honey can be used), syrups, jams, jellies, preserves, jello, etc. Fructose indulgence leads to reactive hypoglycemia. Honey has small amounts of vitamins and minerals, but it affects the body just like refined sugar.

### Pastries

Pies, cakes, any sweetened desserts and jello, which is only sweetened, colored and flavored water with a small amount of gelatin (a highly refined protein). Learn to make your own pies and cakes healthfully from a good cookbook using no concentrated foods.

### Cheese

Cheese is not a good food. It is made by a putrefactive process which results in the production of amines, ammonia, irritating fatty

143

acids (butyric, caprylic, etc.) and lactic acid. These are all waste products which cause irritation to nerves and to the gastrointestinal tract. Tyramine, one of the toxic amines produced in cheese, may cause migraine headache. Certain of the amines can interact with the nitrates present in the stomach to form nitrosamine, a cancer-producing agent.

An intolerance to lactose, the chief carbohydrate of cheese and milk, is probably the most common food sensitivity in America. Rennet, an enzyme, is used in the curdling of milk for cheese manufacture. Most rennet is obtained from the whole stomach lining of calves, kids, or pigs, and a varying percentage from vegetable sources.

A recent study showed elevated blood sugars overnight in well-controlled diabetic who ate pizza only for supper. When they ate the same number of calories, but no cheese products, their blood sugars remained normal overnight.[70]

## Refined Grains

White bread, buns, melba toast, crackers and saltines, cakes, cookies, white macaroni and spaghetti, white rice, bolted cornmeal, cream of wheat and other refined grain products. Make your own whole grain melba toast and melba waffles. (See recipes in *Eat For Strength.*) Crackers, cakes and cookies are unhealthful if made with baking soda or powder, eggs, milk, shortening and most flavorings and colorings. They can, however, be made healthful. The whole grain pastas require a little more cooking, but with a bit of experience the cook handles these just as well as boxed cereals.

## Sweet Fruits and Vegetables

All dried fruits (raisins, dates, figs, etc.) are concentrated foods. It is easy to overeat them, overloading the body with too much food. Having overworked the digestive system most people will experience an "all gone" feeling before the next meal. This sensation results from fatigue of the digestive organs. Bananas, mangoes, watermelon (difficult for some to digest) and sweet potatoes should be avoided by most patients for at least one month, because they are too sweet. Grapes, if eaten generously, may cause shakiness or weakness before the next meal.

### Caffeine Drinks

Coffee (even Sanka and Decaff), tea, cola drinks, and chocolate.   Tea and cocoa products cause constipation.  All members of this food group cause problems for hypoglycemics and diabetics. Accelerated aging, the risk of different cancers and heart disease are all increased by the use of these products.

### Tobacco

Nicotine has been recognized as a cause of hypoglycemia. It is a potent stimulator of insulin production leading to the entire syndrome of high insulin levels followed by disease. Tobacco must be strictly avoided.

### Alcohol

Alcohol is also highly injurious. It is a concentrated carbohydrate, a pancreatic stimulant and toxin and a cellular poison. Even small amounts accelerate aging.

### Soft Drinks

All kinds, including *Kool-Aid*, bottled drinks, etc. Fruit juices may on occasion be used as part of the fluid in some recipes, but generally water is better.  Fruit juices should not be taken regularly at meals in large quantities as they interfere with digestion, dump quickly into the bloodstream and displace other, more important foods.  Perhaps two or three ounces could be sipped slowly at an occasional meal.  Never use any beverage between meals except water and clear, unsweetened herb tea.

### Condiments

Spices have a number of harmful influences on the body and nervous system.  In India, Mexico and Korea there is a high incidence of cancer of the esophagus and stomach due to the heavy use of spices.  Many spices are capable of causing distortions of mental functioning and poor concentration.

Vinegar, even that labeled apple cider vinegar, is irritating to the nervous system and to body tissues. Pickles may be prepared from a good recipe, being essentially canned cucumbers with lemon juice and salt. (See *Eat For Strength* for the method.) All products made with vinegar such as pickles and pickle relish, mustard, catsup, hot pepper sauce, commercial mayonnaise and other products must be avoided. Read labels and look for recipes for easy to make substitutes.

### Medicines Containing Caffeine

Anacin, A.P.C., B.C., Caffergot, Cope, Coricidin, Dolor, Empirin Compound, Excedrin, Fiorinal, 4-Way Cold Tablets, Stanback, Trigesic, Vanquish and others.

## Some General Principles

When you eat is just as important as what you eat. Eat a substantial breakfast and lunch. Supper, if eaten, should be only whole grains or fruit. We have found that the **two-meal plan** allows the body the greatest opportunity for recovery from the heavy work of digestion. (Insulin-dependent diabetics should almost always eat three meals a day as previously noted. Occasionally in difficult to control cases, a bed-time snack may also be necessary.)

A good **schedule for meals** is approximately 7:00a.m. for breakfast and 2:00p.m. for lunch. Drink only beverage tea for supper. Your body needs rest for greater healing, and the hours when this is best accomplished are between the hours of 3:00p.m. through 5:00a.m. Optimum healing can be accomplished only if your body is not exhausting itself by digesting food after 3:00p.m. Get to bed on time and get up on time 365 days a year. Set your schedule and stick to it. Be sure to keep a window open for fresh air in your bedroom, even a small opening in the winter, because morning headaches often occur from stale air.

The reason the hypoglycemic syndrome has developed is because the **pancreas is overworked**. This small organ needs as much rest as possible. Two meals per day rather than three, allows the pancreas an extra opportunity to recover. Although we are accustomed to eating three meals per day, a third meal forces the pancreas to work hard once again, when it could be resting and recovering.

Allowing **five hours to pass between meals** is also important. This length of time provides at least one hour for the "interdigestive phase." During this phase some necessary housekeeping occurs--cleansing the intestinal wall and lining, recharging the products needed for digestion and resetting the nervous mechanism controlling the movement of the bowel.

Those who do not get at least an hour for the **interdigestive phase** have more gastritis, peptic ulcers, small bowel disease, colon polyps and diverticula and even cancer of the colon.

Do not vary mealtimes, even by as little as a few minutes, until your health recovery is complete. Even then strive to **be regular** in all your habits. It pays large dividends.

Drink **no fluids with meals**, but be sure to drink at least eight glasses (eight ounces each) of liquids between meals, beginning no sooner than one hour after eating. Drink enough water to keep the urine colorless.

**Eating behavior** is related to Type II diabetes in some people. In those with shorter eating times there is greater blood sugar fluctuation. **Hasty eaters** also show greater body weight fluctuation than those who eat slowly. **Chewing** your food well and taking small bites helps to regulate weight and blood sugar. **Peptic ulcers** occur more often in people who do not chew their food well. A buffer substance is produced only with well-chewed meals. A part of the treatment of every diabetic should be instruction on eating slowly.[71]

Many physicians advise a **"high protein"** feeding between meals, a bedtime snack and even eating during the night. This practice will sometimes please the patient, but shows a lack of understanding of the relationship between nutrition and body requirements and will prolong the problem. The pancreas, which has been overstimulated by too many meals and too much food, needs rest for recovery. It should be stimulated only at certain specified intervals so that it can regain its rhythmical pattern. Mealtimes should be regular, with as little change in schedule as possible. Nothing should be eaten between meals!

Insure an adequate supply of **magnesium** in the diet. If signs occur of a deficiency such as irregular heartbeats, low calcium in the blood or muscle jerks, a supplement may be needed for a few weeks. Epsom salts, 1-2 teaspoons per day in water should be adequate. Try not to use too much so that diarrhea is caused. Restoring the level of magnesium will often greatly reduce the amount of insulin needed.[72]

**Diabetic children** tend to have lower blood magnesium levels and lower bone densities than normal children. When magnesium is low, calcium and potassium are also usually low. The key to calcium and potassium levels is magnesium, not supplements with calcium and potassium. Correct the magnesium level and the other two minerals will normalize. A low level of either calcium or potassium is a clue that magnesium is low.

### *How To Deal With A Sinking Feeling Without Eating*

1. Determine that "thou shalt not eat." There are ways of dealing with this problem without eating, since eating between meals delays healing and does further damage.

2. Much of that "all gone" feeling is from acute fluid shifts, not from a drop in blood sugar. Drinking an eight ounce glass of water every 10 minutes for an hour, will do wonders for the sensation.

3. Lie down for a few minutes and breathe deeply and very slowly, about five breaths per minute. The sinking feeling and tremulousness will pass quickly. As soon as it passes, get up and have faith that the retraining of your liver and pancreas through the recovery program will work to keep you on your feet.

### *Other Things to Know*

Two important preventive factors for Type I diabetes are: first, take regular **exercise.** The second factor is to avoid cow's milk throughout life. The protein in cow's milk may trigger Type I diabetes in susceptible children.[73]

Women are especially at risk for diabetes if they smoke. The risk rises with the **number of cigarettes** smoked. A study of 114,247 women showed that those smoking 25 cigarettes or more each day have almost twice the risk of diabetes as non-smokers.[74]

When appetite gets "out of control" in the hypoglycemic, the result is not simply feeling bad for a few hours. It may require several weeks to regain a sense of well-being after just a short period of indiscretion. Some people are highly sensitive to any **transgression of health laws.** Even if no ill effect is immediately felt, the deterioration of vital structures will proceed more rapidly.

We advise that **legumes** (beans, peas, peanuts, etc.) and whole grains such as rice be used as main dishes as often as possible, rather than animal products. These simple and inexpensive foods are excellent sources of protein, and have the advantage of not raising the blood cholesterol or endangering the health with diseases transmitted in animal flesh. They also tend to have about one-third less calories than even the leanest of meats.

**Exercise** is your best friend. It is an essential part of the treatment. Twenty minutes per day is minimal. One hour daily 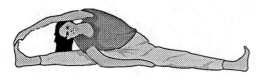 is better, but on certain days three to five hours may be needed. Do not get sunburned and do not make your muscles sore with too much exercise. Both of these are unhealthful. Build to a good exercise level gradually. Rushing makes muscles sore and is not a healthful practice. Exercise helps keep your appetite under control, neutralizes stress, lowers blood cholesterol, promotes digestion, lowers the cancer risk, reduces high blood pressure and normalizes blood sugar. Make it your daily companion. Breathe deeply while exercising and meditate on nature as you work out.

There is no need to lose confidence in the doctor who is treating you; he or she is doing the very best they know. Metabolic and nutritional problems are still poorly understood by most physicians. A patient may need a physician in other ways, and you should not be needlessly cut off from him or her.

## *Occupation*

Another subject of great concern which needs to be discussed is how you make your living. If your occupation is overly stressful for you, it will be to your benefit if you begin to think about whether the stress, and/or the money (no matter how much money you may be making) is worth losing your health over. Many people who are unhappy and pressured with their work situation will develop diabetes because of the stress on the pancreas. Along with the diabetes come all the complications of heart disease and other problems. If the way you make a living is killing you, it may be necessary to alter your work situation or to look into the possibilities of a new career.

As a concluding word, be aware that if you or someone you know is struggling with hypoglycemia, the symptoms include being nervous, irritable, a tendency to get neurotic or self-centered, to brood over supposed ills and to dwell on physical or emotional symptoms. Be gentle with yourself and others and expect recovery.

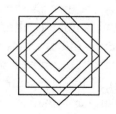

# CHAPTER TEN

# Weight Control, Hypertension, Stress Control, and Causes of Insulin Resistance

## WEIGHT CONTROL

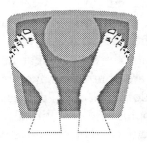

In almost all cases of Type II diabetes, control of the disease is completely determined by control of appetite, weight and exercise.

There are certain measures that can be taken to insure weight loss and control. Although they may be difficult to accustom yourself to, they become easier with practice. Don't worry about the reactions of your family and friends. After they understand what you are doing and why, most likely they will support your efforts. If anyone questions what you are doing, say, "Doctor's Orders."

Most of the time, it is better to prepare your own meals and eat at home or bring your meal with you to work or wherever you go. If you plan to eat in a restaurant, call ahead and make sure they are agreeable to preparing a meal the way you need to eat it. Today, many restaurants have vegetarian entrees, but you must still be aware of what they put in or on top of these dishes. Many restaurants will leave the fatty sauces off your vegetables. You can bring your own condiments; most restaurant owners will not object. Also, there are many health food restaurants which are so health-conscious you may be able to order a meal without asking for any alterations. But do ask questions if you are unsure and don't eat anything if you don't know what is in it. You'll get used to this kind of behavior and you'll feel better for it. (See Chapter Nine for foods allowed and foods to avoid.)

If you are invited for dinner at a private home, explain your situation and ask if the hostess would feel comfortable and is it acceptable for you to bring your own food if necessary. The other person will understand when you explain you are on a health recovery diet which does not include fats and sugars.

### Set Points For Weight Control

Set points are established markers for body processes. We have many hundreds of set points in the body, from the length hair will grow before it falls out to how high blood proteins are. The body's metabolic processes defend individual set points and resist altering them. But once a set point has been breached, there may be rapid and significant changes in weight until a new set point is established. This new set point can be higher or lower than before. There are controlling factors which cause the set point to go up or down. We will discuss those factors which make the set point slide continually upward, so that you may alter these factors and bring your set point down.

### Factors That Affect Set Points

(+) indicates raising the set point, (-) indicates lowering it.
1. The amount and type of dietary fats (+) Saturated fat, generally animal fat, will raise the set point more than unsaturated fat from plant sources
2. Eating between meals (+)

3. Regular, moderate exercise  (-)
4. Sedentary lifestyle  (+)
5. Irregular meal times  (+)
6. Eating of sweets  (+)
7. Loss of sleep  (+)
8. Green, leafy vegetables and salads  (-)
9. Late and heavy suppers  (+)
10. Eating many varieties at one meal  (+)
11. Protein of animal origin  (+)

*Weight Control Guidelines*
   The following is a set of guidelines for planning your program of weight loss and weight control. If you observe these suggestions you will bring the set point down for weight, which will reduce your weight, blood sugar and cholesterol.
   1. Cut out all free fats completely. This includes butter, margarine, mayonnaise, fried foods, cooking fats, salad oils, peanut butter and all other nut or seed butters.
   2. You need to consider becoming a total vegetarian. When the Lord made food, he made certain foods that are produced by animals, like milk from mother animals, to make baby animals grow. Milk, cheese, butterfat, cottage cheese, cream cheese, yogurt and buttermilk all make animals grow. If the animal is full-grown and continues to eat milk and milk products, it can grow fat. These products make human beings grow also, and many adults who still use milk products, will grow fat. Since these foods were not formulated for the human body by the Designer, they cause many malfunctions in our body machinery by throwing our chemical make-up into a state of imbalance.
      When we are young, animal products make us grow quickly, but they predispose us to many illnesses such as allergies, colds, sore throats, earaches and digestive complaints, even though we seem to be

healthy. When we get older these products cause us to grow fat and the damage caused by them becomes expressed as hypertension, overweight, diabetes, cancer or heart disease. No animal product - meat, milk, eggs or cheese - is essential for good nutrition. While these products contain essential nutrients, these essential nutrients can be obtained in many other types of foods.

3. Eat nothing after three in the afternoon. The metabolism changes at about that time and food taken after 3:00 p.m. makes the set point increase. Drinking herb teas as desired is permissible after three. If you need to be sociable in a group, pour yourself a cup of herbal tea and sip it while enjoying the company of your friends. Carry tea bags with you for emergency use. Never eat a morsel, not even a bite of celery, between meals or after 3:00 p.m.

4. The more raw foods you eat, the better it will be for weight loss. Try going for a period of 30 days in which you eat nothing but raw foods.

   It is necessary to go through a transition phase before you attempt to eat a totally raw food diet. Your system is mainly used to digesting cooked foods, and a sudden change to all raw foods could cause minor to severe digestive problems. Slowly increase the quantity of raw foods you are now eating. If your breakfast menu is hot cereal, add several raw fruits. If your dinner menu is cooked grains, beans and vegetables, try eating your vegetables raw instead. Give yourself at least one month to gradually work into a raw food diet.

   Some people will experience digestive problems with raw food, even if they have faithfully followed a transitional diet. This is attributed to individual digestive strengths and weaknesses and the physical condition in general. If you notice symptoms beginning to appear such as abdominal pain, gas, bloating, constipation or diarrhea, try making raw fruit or vegetable juices with a juicer. Store-bought juices will give less benefits. They are no longer fresh and have lost many of their nutrients during shipping and storage. Juices should be sipped at the beginning of meals and sipped slowly to mix with saliva. Sip fruit juice before a fruit meal and vegetable juice before a vegetable meal.

You can also make fruit or vegetable purees in a blender. A vegetable puree can be warmed slightly and enjoyed as a thick broth. By using juices and purees, you will still obtain the benefits of raw foods but you will experience less or no digestive upsets.

Breakfast can be fruit in any form - dried, canned without sugar, frozen or fresh - with up to 1/4 cup of nuts or seeds. For lunch try any kind of vegetables in the quantity you desire, along with corn on the cob or whole kernel corn. Limit the variety of foods to no more than four; two or three is better. An example of a delicious, well-balanced lunch is: A large bed of shredded cabbage, finely grated rutabaga, carrot juice with the pulp mixed back in (not the juice alone) and 1/4 to 1/3 cup of shredded unsweetened coconut. Green peas fresh or frozen or any frozen vegetables (small raw okra is especially good), freshly juiced carrots or beets with the pulp added back to the juice and raw sunflower seeds, make a delightful salad. Squeeze a few drops of lemon juice on it and a sprinkle of dry or fresh mint leaves or sweet basil. This salad would constitute your entire meal.

A fruit salad can be made with apples, oranges and sunflower seeds. You may have any kind of raw nuts, but limit the portion to the 1/4 to 1/2 cup quantity. Certain nuts have more fat than others and it is better to cut down on the fattier ones. The following nuts and seeds are listed from high fat to low fat content: cashew, pecan, macadamia, sesame, walnut, almond, coconut, pistachio, sunflower, flax, pumpkin, chest-nut.

5. Immediately after meals take some exercise out-of-doors for about 25 minutes. It should not be strenuous, but should be brisk or vigorous. Walking, yard work, bicycling, etc., will all suffice. Be sure not to exercise to the point that you hinder digestion.

6. The smaller the variety of food eaten at one meal, the lower the set point for weight. More weight will be gained from a 600 calorie meal containing ten different dishes made from complex recipes, than a 600 calorie meal containing only two or three simple dishes plus bread and      spread. The smaller variety is also beneficial for digestion and health of insulin receptors.

## *Method of Fasting*

Fasting was discussed in Chapter Two. An easy method of fasting is repeated here. Fasting is a beneficial way to gain appetite control, help accustom yourself to the tastes of different foods, restore function of insulin receptors and to help lose weight.

Fasting can be done easily by omitting supper on day one and all meals on day two. On day three, the fast can be broken by eating one-quarter the size of the usual breakfast, one-half the usual lunch and no supper. On day four, three-quarters of the usual breakfast can be eaten. Lunch on day four will be the first full meal after the fast. Spend as many days breaking the fast as were spent in the fast.

## *Rule of Thumb For Average Weight*

For the average American, a rule of thumb to calculate your weight is as follows: Give yourself 100 pounds for your first five feet in height. Then add five pounds per inch thereafter if you are a woman, and 6 to 7 if you are a man, depending on how muscular you are.

When a person is fighting a disease, it is beneficial to be on the thin side. We suggest about 5% below the average American weight for those with serious diseases such as diabetes.

## How to Bring the Blood Pressure Down

Reactions to various physical and emotional influences in life may cause the blood pressure to rise. These influences 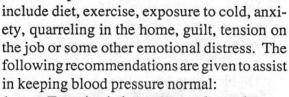 include diet, exercise, exposure to cold, anxiety, quarreling in the home, guilt, tension on the job or some other emotional distress. The following recommendations are given to assist in keeping blood pressure normal:

1.      Exercise is important to keep the blood vessels in a healthy tone, equalizing the "tensions" between the autonomic (automatic) and somatic (under conscious control) divisions of the nervous system, and in clearing the blood of excessive fats or sugars. Do some useful labor, such as gardening or yard work, at a moderate pace for about one hour each day. The pace should be what is described as "vigorous but not violent." Outdoor labor is usually more beneficial than indoor labor. Even the sense of satisfaction in work well done is stabilizing to the blood pressure.

2. Run in place for six minutes twice daily to reduce the blood pressure.

3. Starting with the muscles of the legs, thighs and back, tense the muscles as much as possible and hold for several seconds. Gradually relax. Next, tense the abdomen, chest, arms, neck and head, hold for a few seconds, then relax. Use this routine twice a day.

4. For a natural tranquilizer, take a long walk at a rapid pace to use up excess nervous energy. Read the next section on stress.

5. Practice a deep breathing exercise three times daily. The deep breathing exercise consists of taking very deep breaths held to the count of twenty, exhaling and holding to the count of ten. This can be done while driving. Repeat twenty to sixty times.

6. Five important pointers to remember about diet are: First, use a diet such as the "Calming Diet," outlined under Stress Control in the following section. Second, use few concentrated foods such as animal products, fats, sweets, meat substitutes or concentrated proteins. Eat non-concentrated foods such as fruits, vegetables and whole grains freely. Third, to prevent high blood pressure, do not use more than one-half to one teaspoon of salt per day. It may be necessary to totally eliminate all salt and sodium products for a while. Baking soda and baking powder are also high in sodium as well as being unhealthful in other ways. All baked goods using these substances should be avoided. After high blood pressure has developed, salt, baking soda, baking powder, most antacids, even toothpaste and all other sources of sodium may need to be eliminated for a time until the blood pressure is entirely normal and stable. Do not forget that sodium is in many over-the-counter and prescription drugs. Fourth, free fats promote high blood pressure. Free fats are listed in the weight control section. Fifth, the diet must be constructed to reduce the weight, if weight is above the ideal.

*Ways to Perk Up Salt-free Foods*

To perk up foods which taste dull without salt, try using herbs. Basil should be tried with a number of different dishes, both fruit and vegetable, as it goes well with many flavors. Use dill on vegetables, potatoes, rice, macaroni and potato salad. Mint is good with beans, rice, vegetable soups, pumpkin and squash dishes, and can be used in fruit salads and carob desserts. Chives perk up potatoes and salads. Rosemary can be used on rice dishes, pastas, potatoes and wheat dishes. Oregano goes well with pastas, salads and on broccoli. Cilantro is delightful in any salad. Grow your own fresh herbs in pots inside your home for these delicious flavors. You will find picking them fresh gives a surprisingly special flavor to your dishes.

7. A program to reduce blood pressure should begin with a day of fasting, followed by three days in which only apples are eaten (raw, cooked, stewed, dried or frozen) at each of three meals. Then for the following two days eat only fruit and salt-free, whole grain bread or cereal for breakfast and vegetables and salt-free bread or rice for dinner. Eat only one apple for supper. (Omit supper if overweight.)

8. Careful attention to proper clothing of the extremities is essential to calm the autonomic nervous system and to equalize the circulation. Cool skin causes an alarm reaction in the autonomic nerves.

9. For patients who can tolerate it, the "short cold hip bath" is beneficial. For the first treatment, start with water temperature at 85 to 88 degrees. The patient sits with only the hips in a tub of water for three to three and a half minutes. Reduce the water temperature about five degrees each time the bath is taken until a temperature of 65 degrees is achieved. Repeat the bath daily as needed. There is an initial elevation of blood pressure of five to 15 points when the bath begins, but soon the blood pressure begins to drop.

10. A neutral bath for ten to 30 minutes at the end of the day in a tub of water that feels neither warm nor cool (92 to 96 degrees) can have a remarkably calming effect and often lowers blood pressure. After the bath, cool the body gradually while lying well-covered in bed. After thirty minutes, when sweating has stopped, take a regular shower, rub dry vigorously with a coarse towel and dress in dry clothes.

11. Certain herbs are very helpful for bringing the blood pressure down. Watermelon Seed tea acts as a diuretic. Make this tea by grinding one teaspoon of the seed in a seed mill or blender. Boil one cup of water, turn flame off, add tea and steep for 20-30 minutes. Strain and drink. Other diuretic teas are Buchu, Burdock, Dandelion and Cornsilk. One teaspoon of only one of these or one teaspoon of each, if needed, is added to one cup of water. This may be drunk as often as every two hours if needed, except for the Burdock, of which only four cups per day should be taken.

    Hawthorn Berry and Dandelion used together are excellent for blood pressure. Use one teaspoon of each to one cup boiling water, turn flame off, steep 20-30 minutes, strain and drink four to eight cups per day.

12. During each moment that your mind is not occupied with active labor or social discourse, practice concentrating on certain virtues (love, joy, peace, patience, goodness, meekness, faith, etc.), and the attributes of God (His eternalness, faithfulness, honesty, loving-kindness, creativity, intelligence, etc.)

## *Hypertension and Stress Control*

Paradoxically, not only overwork and a frenzy of activity, but too much leisure can cause stress. Certain conditions of the mind can also cause stress. Jealousy, being unappreciated, a lack of genuine religion, anticipating future wants and stimulating amusements all cause stress. You can control stress if you approach the stressor correctly. First, face your most unpleasant stressor, then examine, review and discuss it in your mind. You may wish to take notes on your thoughts. Make an immediate plan to reduce that stressor to manageable proportions. And since physical factors can also be an important aspect of stress, put the following program into practice:

1. Observe strict regularity for meals, taking no food or drink between meals. Omit all evening food, retiring only after digestion is complete.
2. Guard against overeating or undereating. Stress mounts after too much food.
3. Use a "Calming Diet," containing no nerve stimulating or irritating foods such as hot pepper, ginger, cinnamon, cloves, nutmeg, vinegar or anything made with vinegar such as pickles, mayonnaise, catsup, mustard, etc.. Avoid foods having a fermenting, putrefying or rotting phase of processing such as sauerkraut, cheese, soy sauce and similar products. Abstain from baking soda and baking powder products, caffeine and other methyl xanthines such as theophylline and theobromine which are found in coffee, tea, colas, chocolate and nicotine. Eliminate all concentrated foods such as wheat germ, margarine, dried skim milk and all animal products. Take plenty of raw fruits, vegetables, whole grains and legumes. Use nuts sparingly.
4. Eliminate sugar, honey, coconut, dried or very sweet fruits and vegetables during periods when you feel stressed.
5. Eat freely of foods that are high in B-vitamins, such as greens, legumes and whole grains. The B-vitamins are called "good disposition vitamins."
6. Stimulate the skin by brushing the body with a stiff brush before a daily cool shower. Alternate a hot and cold water spray over the adrenal areas of the back at the end of each bath or shower. Use about 20-30 seconds for the hot and ten seconds for the cold for five exchanges.
7. Be regular in bedtime, arising time, elimination, study periods, etc. Regularity in all things is essential.
8. Take a sunbath daily, weather permitting, fully clothed if you desire and early in the morning (before 10:00), or late in the afternoon (after 3:00). Sit or lie in the

sun in clothing appropriate for the weather (warm woolens in the winter and cool cottons in the summer), protecting the eyes from bright rays with a hat or sunglasses.

9. Do deep breathing exercises. Get in fresh air and breathe in and out through the nose 40-50 times.

10. Take a brisk walk holding your head up, with a cheerful expression on your face, breathing deeply and with good posture. Walk in nature an hour or more each day. Pay close attention to things of nature as you walk - a countless array of plants, animals, rocks and many other things have been provided by a loving Creator to attract our minds from self to Himself.

11. Start a graduated exercise program. Gardening with bare feet and hands in the soil may be helpful to some. Exercise neutralizes stress.

12. Check transit time; the length of time your intestinal tract requires to process two teaspoons of moistened sesame seed, from the hour you take them until the last of the marker appears in the stool. Up to twenty-eight hours is a normal transit time.

13. Have laboratory work done. Have tests for blood sugar levels, Hematocrit (red blood cell test) and T-4 (thyroid).

14. Control talking carefully: not too much, not too little and only about cheerful subjects; not about self or a single subject. This is important.

15. Take a neutral bath (described in number ten of How to Bring the Blood Pressure Down) daily or more often.

16. Develop a daily program of Bible study and prayer. Learn to control thoughts and to dwell on heavenly themes.

## *Exercises For Gangrenous Feet*

While seated, try to make every foot movement your condition will allow you to make - point the toe up, then down, to the right, then to the left and stretch the heel as if pressing it into an imaginary pillow.

If your condition allows it, stand on your tiptoes for five seconds, then alternate feet and stand on tiptoe for two seconds with each foot individually. If this exercise agrees with you, build up the time day by day until you have added ten seconds to each exercise.

We have found our patients receive benefit from walking as well as from stretching. If the feet are swollen, a pair of inexpensive canvas shoes may be cut in appropriate places to relieve pressure. Use care to prevent any kind of trauma to the feet, including sunburn or pressure blisters, as these problems may never heal and could force an amputation.

## Chronic Dehydration Plays A Role in Diabetes

Acute dehydration and chronic dehydration which has resulted in a "new steady state" of water metabolism can both cause disease. Yet most people are unaware that any problem exists if thirst does not reach annoying levels.

Every organ and tissue, from the joints to the brain, are injured to some degree by dehydration. Cleansing of tissues is impeded, joints are not lubricated, lenses in the eyes can start forming cataracts, allergenic substances can concentrate to the point they cause asthma or hay fever, the lungs can release histamine because of concentrated blood and the metabolism is altered in many ways that involve the pancreas.

Overeating results in a condition of the blood which is essentially the same as dehydration. Dehydration triggers the production of prostaglandin, a hormone which reduces insulin production and increases water movement to the pancreatic cells. Overeating results in insulin inhibition just at a time it is needed most.[75]

### Signs of Dehydration

You can tell when you are likely to be dehydrated by the following signs:

1. Ask yourself about your previous 48 hour history of

water drinking - has it been adequate? Six to 10 glasses per day are needed.

2.  Check your heart rate - is it above the usual rate? This is one of the earliest signs of dehydration.
3.  Are your skin and mucous membranes dry? Are your lips chapped?
4.  When the blood is pressed out of the skin of your abdomen is there a delay for the blood to run back in again? If 2-3 seconds elapse, there is significant water loss.
5.  Is there mottling or coolness of the skin of your extremities? These indicate circulation retardation in the part involved.
6.  Has there been disturbance of the nervous system - poor attention focus, lethargy with hyperirritability to touching, sounds or bright lights in the room?[76]

## Causes of Insulin Resistance

A large percentage of people with diabetes, high blood pressure and coronary heart disease are found to be insulin resistant. Insulin resistance has been shown to be the initiating factor in these diseases. The tendency to be insulin resistant is inherited, and will also be seen among family members. Yet there are lifestyle factors which influence insulin resistance and the development of these diseases.

In order for insulin to be useful to us, we must have insulin receptors on body cells. If these receptors (which accept insulin united with sugar and carry them both into the cell--sugar alone will not be accepted) are reduced in number, sugar cannot get into cells, and instead stays in the blood stream. This makes blood sugar rise.

What factors cause insulin receptors to be reduced and insulin resistance to develop? Known factors are as follows:

1.  Overeating
2.  Use of alcohol
3.  Overuse of sugar
4.  Overweight

5. Habitually eating too great a variety of food at one meal
6. Overuse of very concentrated foods
7. Eating between meals
8. Late night meals
9. Use of meat, milk, eggs and cheese

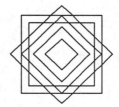

# CHAPTER ELEVEN

# Listings of Food Sources Containing Essential Nutrients, Menus, Recipes

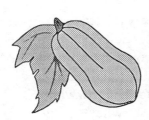 It is important to remember that diabetes and hypoglycemia are total nutrient disorders. It is not possible to add only a certain "healthy" food to your diet, instead of correcting your entire menu, and expect to experience improved health. All of the nutrients we have spoken about which have a beneficial effect on diabetic and hypoglycemic conditions, work in harmony with one another. These nutrients can be found in larger quantities in specific foods. These foods, when emphasized, in combination with a vegetarian diet that includes unrefined grains and no meat or animal products, will help the body establish a normal supply of essential nutrients. This balance will be reflected as enhanced health.

The following is a list of several important nutrients and the foods in which they may be found. These are specifically beneficial to diabetics.

1. Magnesium. Activator of enzymes and necessary for regulation of temperature, synthesis of protein, contraction of muscles, normal bowel action, normal heart function, blood pressure regulation, transmission of nerve impulses and thought processes. Magnesium is found in whole grains, cashews, almonds, seeds, soy and black beans, raw green leafy vegetables, corn, avocados, butternut squash, carob flour, figs, cantaloupes, bananas, apples, peaches and lemons.

2. Manganese. Associated with good glucose tolerance, effective enzyme activity, healthy neurological processes and digestion and appropriate control of fats. Manganese is found in whole grains, nuts, dry beans, leafy green vegetables, oranges and blueberries.

3. Chromium. Necessary for carbohydrate metabolism, utilization of sugars, hormone and enzyme functions and helps to regulate cholesterol. Chromium is found in whole grains, brewer's yeast [77] and in small quantities in many vegetables.

4. Myo-inositol. A muscle sugar, closely related to glucose. Improves nerve function and is helpful in alleviating diabetic neuropathy. It is stored in the brain, heart and skeletal muscles. Myo-inositol is found in peanuts, cantaloupes, grapefruits and all citrus, whole grains, beans and legumes, yeast, wheat germ, blackstrap molasses and nuts.

   Diabetics somehow lose large amounts of myo-inositol in the urine. It promotes body production of lecithin, which is a part of nerve cells. This may account for the nerve involvement in diabetics. Coffee and its brown beverage relatives (tea, colas and chocolate) deplete the body stores of myo-inositol. [78]

5. Vanadium. A trace mineral that helps bring blood sugar back to normal. Vanadium is found in whole

grains, white potatoes, carrots, radishes, white cabbage, onions, string beans, cucumbers, avocados, blueberries, apples, pears, bananas, prunes and plums.
6. Zinc. Component of insulin. Promotes mental alertness. Whole grains, brewer's yeast, raw seeds-especially pumpkin seeds, popcorn and legumes are very high in zinc.
7. Vitamin B-12. B-12 deficiency in the body is a very rare disorder and the overwhelming majority of cases occur in non-vegetarians. Known causes of B-12 depletion are a lack of hydrochloric acid in the stomach, the removal or disease of the ileum, competition for B-12 by microorganisms or intestinal parasites and toxic substances in the body. B-12 is naturally produced in the body in the teeth, gums, tonsils, tongue, nasopharynx, conjunctiva of the eyes, esophagus and upper stomach. Reported food sources of B-12 include wheat, soybeans, olives, fruits, tomatoes, cabbage, celery, kale, turnip greens, broccoli, leeks and alfalfa. Most authorities doubt whether B-12 is consistently present in plant sources. If present, it is in very minute quantities, and even its presence is variable.
8. Fiber. Improves intestinal action, ties up toxins and some excess sugar and reduces cholesterol. Fiber is found in fruits, vegetables, beans, nuts and seeds. All animal products are entirely devoid of fiber.

## Elimination and Challenge Diet

The elimination and challenge diet should be used *if symptoms* of hypoglycemia *have not diminished* after following the Health Recovery Program for one year. This hanging on of symptoms may indicate food allergies. (See next page for foods to avoid on Elimination and Challenge Diet.)

## Foods to Avoid in Elimination and Challenge Diet:

Dairy products (account for
over 60% of food allergies)
Chocolate
Colas
Coffee
Tea
Eggs
Pork
Beef
Fish
Legumes - Peanuts - Soybean
products
Citrus fruits and juices
Tomatoes - Potatoes - Eggplant
Peppers - Tobacco also
Corn - Cornstarch - Corn products
Wheat
Oatmeal
Yeast
Cane Sugar
Cinnamon - irritating
substances, spices
Beer, Alcohol
Artificial food colors
Strawberries
Apples
Bananas
Nuts - all kinds
Seeds
Lettuce
Garlic
Onion
Rice

## Foods Allowed:

Grains: Barley, Buckwheat,
Millet, Rye
Thickeners: Tapioca,
Arrowroot
Herbs: Basil, Bayleaf, Dill,
Parsley, Sage, Thyme

Vegetables: Artichoke,
Asparagus, Avocado,
Broccoli, Cabbage,
Cauliflower, Collards,
Beets, Brussels Sprouts,
Carrots, Celery,
Cucumber, Kale,
Okra, Olives, Rhubarb,
Rutabaga, Spinach,
Squash (Acorn, Butternut,
Hubbard, Summer, Zucchini)
Sweet Potatoes, Swiss Chard,
Turnips

Fruits: Apricot,
Avocado, Blackberries,
Cantaloupe, Figs,
Grapes, Honeydew,
Kiwi, Mango,
Nectarine, Papaya,
Peach, Persimmon,
Pear, Pineapple,
Plums, Pomegranate,
Raspberries,
Watermelon

Dried Fruits: Currants,
Dates, Figs, Pineapple,
Prunes, Raisins

# Menus and Recipes for Health Recovery Program

Now that you have a better idea of what, when and how to eat, you need to know how to prepare these delicious, healthful foods. If you take a little extra time to become familiar with the cooking methods, you can create appetizing meals that will satisfy, nourish and assist you in recovering your health.

Here are several recipes that appear in the meal planner that follows this section. The complete list, and other meal planners may be found in *Eat For Strength*, Oil-Free edition.

### Corn Tamale Pie

| | |
|---|---|
| 1 c. corn meal | ¹/₂ c. Tomato Sauce or 3 c. |
| 2 ¹/₂ c. water | canned tomatoes, and |
| 2 c. whole kernel corn | omit the 2 ¹/₂ c. water |
| ³/₄ c. chopped olives | 1 t. salt or Chicken-Style |
| 1 c. chopped onion | seasoning from the |
| 1 c. chopped green pepper, opt. | health food store |
| ³/₄ c. cold water | |

Bring the water or juice drained from the canned tomatoes to a boil. Blend the corn meal with the cold water. Add the corn meal and salt to the boiling water and stir until it returns to a boil. Let it boil rapidly until it begins to thicken. Reduce heat to low and let simmer for 20-40 minutes. 20 minutes is the minimum time-40 minutes is better. Simmer remaining ingredients in a little bit of water until the onion begins to be transparent. Combine all ingredients. Bake at 350 degrees for 1 hour. Serves 4.

### Oat Waffles

| | |
|---|---|
| 8 c. rolled oats | 2 t. salt |
| 8 c. water | |

Put oats in a baking pan and dextrinize them in the oven at 325 degrees for 5 to 15 minutes, watching carefully so they lightly brown but do not burn. (Dextrinization is the changing of carbohydrates from long chain molecules, as in starches, to shorter chains as in dextrins, by heating. The more these chains are broken down, the more digestible the food becomes. This process also makes grains taste sweeter.) Mix all ingredients together and allow to stand overnight in the refrigerator. Preheat waffle iron but do not allow to smoke. Use 1-1 ½ cups of batter for each waffle. Bake each waffle 12 to 15 minutes before opening waffle iron. Place on bare oven rack at 175 degrees to keep hot until serving time, or cool and freeze for storage. Be certain waffles are nicely browned, as inadequately cooked grains are not as digestible as fully cooked grains.

## Spanish Rice

1 c. cooked garbanzos
3 c. cooked brown rice
½ c. onion
½ c. green pepper
½ t. onion salt

¾ c. tomato paste or cooked
   tomatoes
2 c. water
2 T. soy flour

Chop and saute onion and pepper in a little water. Mix last 4 items and stir into onion and pepper. Simmer gently until thickened, about 3-5 minutes. Add rice and garbanzos. Bake in floured casserole for 25 minutes at 350 degrees. Serves 4. Variation: Substitute green peas for part or all of the garbanzos.

## Millet

1 c. millet
4 c. water

¼ c. sesame meal (optional)
1 t. salt

Mix, bring to a boil, then simmer for 2 ½ hours. Can serve with a fruit or vegetable meal.

## Bean Soup

2 c. any dried beans
2 onions
2 carrots or
2 stalks of celery

2 t. salt
2-3 quarts water
2 t. basil

Check the cooking instructions on beans. Most need to be soaked overnight. Lentils can be cooked without soaking. Most beans need to be cooked for 2-4 hours, except garbanzos which may require 6 hours and lentils which cook for 1 hour. Soak beans overnight (except lentils) in cold water, drain, add 2-3 quarts of fresh water and bring to a boil. Simmer 1-6 hours. After simmering, add all the other ingredients, cover tightly and simmer until vegetables are done, adding more water when necessary. May be served at this point, but also very tasty if you strain through a sieve or whiz in blender with a little water. The soup should then be like heavy cream.

## Baked Tofu

4 c. water
2 1/4 c. soy flour
2/3 c. pimentos
2 and 1/2 t. salt

1/2 c. flour
1/3 c. lemon juice
1/4 t. garlic salt (optional)
2 and 1/2 T. food yeast

Place all ingredients in blender and whiz until smooth. Pour into a small, floured loaf pan. Bake 2 hours at 275 degrees. Keep in oven for another hour after turning off. Chill before turning out of pan. Peel off the brown skin on top and trim loaf to shape. Slice or cube for serving. Use for dinners, in soups, salads and sandwiches.

## Zucchini Squash

Shred zucchini finely. Add an equal quantity of chopped onions. Place in deep pot on medium heat. Stir until the heat draws out liquid for steaming. Serve with a small amount of salt.

## Cabbage and Carrots

Chop cabbage finely. Chop carrots in strips or diagonals. Steam together in a small amount of water until tender. Serve with Chee Sauce.

## Chee Sauce

1 c. tomatoes or
1/2 c. pimentos
1 c. water
1/3 c. lemon juice
1 1/2 t. salt

1 t. onion powder (optional)
1/8 t. garlic powder
2 T. sesame seed (optional)
1 T. yeast flakes

Blenderize all ingredients until smooth. Serve over cooked cabbage and carrots, broccoli, potatoes, rice or use over whole grain macaroni as a cheese substitute and in casseroles.

## Zwieback or Melba Toast

Twice baked bread is very digestible. Make some Zwieback from each batch of bread. Place very thin slices directly on the oven rack. Bake at 175-225 degrees until entirely dry and lightly browned. You can also pull chunks of bread off the unsliced loaf and dry these in a pan.

## Sesame Straws

³/₄ c. water                          2 c. whole wheat flour
¹/₂ t. salt                          ¹/₂ c. sesame seeds

Mix ingredients and let rest for 10 minutes. Divide into two parts and roll on an unoiled cookie sheet. Cut into straws 4 inches by ¹/₃ inches. Bake at 250 degrees for 45 minutes. Watch carefully after 20 minutes as oven settings can vary. Makes 100 straws.

## Corn Dodgers

3 c. corn meal                       2 ¹/₈ c. boiling water
³/₄ t. salt                          ¹/₂ c. unsweetened coconut, opt.

Mix and spoon onto floured cookie sheets. Bake at 375 degrees for 30 minutes. Makes 10 dodgers.

## Haystacks

Zwieback, dried toasted            lettuce
    tortillas, or oil-free          olives
    corn chips                      tomatoes
cooked pinto beans                 Chee Sauce
onions

Put the beans and Chee Sauce in separate bowls. Slice the onions, olives, tomatoes and shred the lettuce. Put each in separate serving bowls. Use Zwieback or oil-free chips as the first layer on each person's plate. Top with layers of beans, lettuce, onions, tomatoes, olives and Chee Sauce.

## Chili

4 c. cooked beans                  1 c. bell pepper, chopped
1 c. onion, chopped                2 t. celery salt or other
2 ¹/₂ c. tomatoes                       seasoning salt

Simmer slowly for 45 minutes. Good with rice or burgers or serve in a soup bowl with a dollop of Wheatonnaise.

## Wheatonnaise

1 c. water                               $^1/_4$ c. wheat flour

Whirl in blender. Boil 15-25 minutes, stirring constantly. Cool and return to blender and add:

$^1/_2$ c. raw carrots                    $^1/_2$ c. water
$^1/_2$ t. salt                           1 T. lemon juice
1 clove garlic or
$^1/_2$ small onion

Whiz until smooth.

## Oat Burgers

2 c. cooked oatmeal                       1-2 c. bread crumbs
1 raw potato                             1 t. salt
$^1/_2$ c. onion                          $^1/_2$ t. sage

Grind potato and onion in blender with a little water if needed. Mix with cooked oatmeal. Add remaining items and mix. Use more crumbs if water is used in blender. Form patties and bake at 350 degrees for 30 minutes. Turn patties and bake 15 minutes more, until nicely browned. Serve with Holiday Gravy.

## Holiday Gravy

3 c. water                               1 t. salt or Chicken-
$^1/_2$ c. flour, dextrinized                Style seasoning
1 T. food yeast

Place flour in dry pan in oven at 300 degrees for 10-15 minutes to lightly brown (dextrinize) flour. Barley flour is a good flour to use in gravies to increase the variety of grains used. Barley flour is mild in flavor and light in color. If not commercially available, make flour in blender from pearl barley. Mix all ingredients in a blender and cook in a saucepan, stirring until thickened. Cover and simmer for 15-25 minutes. Serves 8-10.

## Cole Slaw

6 c. shredded cabbage          Soyonnaise

Combine cabbage with enough Soyonnaise to coat lightly.


## Soyonnaise

2 c. hot water                 1 t. salt
2/3 c. Soyagen                 1/2 t. dill weed (optional)
1/2 c. hot rice                1 t. Chicken Style seasoning
1/4 c. lemon juice

Blenderize all ingredients, except lemon juice, until very smooth. Stir in lemon juice. Chill and serve.


## Seasoned Gravy

2 c. water                     1 t. onion powder
1/4 c. whole grain flour       1/4 t. any mixed herbs
1/2 t. salt

Mix all ingredients and cook in saucepan for 10 minutes. Use as stock for stews or serve over vegetarian burgers, potatoes, rice, casseroles and cooked vegetables.


## Hommus (This is a favorite. Try it!)

2 c. cooked garbanzos or green     salt, if needed
   soybeans                        1 T. chopped parsley (optional)
1/2 c. sesame seed                 3 T. lemon juice
1 clove garlic, opt.

Liquefy beans, salt, (1/2 t. if garbanzos are unsalted), garlic and sesame seeds with barely enough bean broth to make blender turn. Sprinkle with garlic powder if garlic clove is omitted. Serve over Zwieback with parsley, as a sandwich spread or filling. Use anywhere you would use mayonnaise - salads, potatoes, rice or as a margarine substitute. 3-4 servings.

## Bean Spread or Gravy

Use any leftover beans. Place 1-2 cups in blender with enough water to make a thick spread consistency. If a gravy is desired, add more water or Soy Milk. Season with onion, garlic, salt and herbs.

## Soy Milk

2 c. water                          1 c. soy flour

Whiz water and flour in blender. Cook for 1-3 hours in double boiler. This is the soy base. Store in refrigerator. To make soy milk, place 1 cup of soy base in blender. Add enough water to make the consistency of milk. Add salt and for a creamier texture, add up to 1 cup of any cooked cereal. To alter flavor, may add and whiz an apple, banana, orange (peeled with seeds removed), vanilla, maple flavoring, etc.

## Millet Pudding

1 c. hot, cooked millet             1 t. vanilla
2 c. pineapple juice                $1/4$ t. salt

Blend smooth, pour into serving dish and chill. Layer or decorate with fruit such as pineapple, bananas, peaches, berries or grapes if desired. Instead of pineapple juice use several ripe bananas.

## Fruited Oats

4 c. boiling water                  $1/4$ c. dates or other dried fruit
1 t. salt                           1 large banana, chopped
1 $3/4$ c. oats

Mix in the order given except for the banana, which is stirred in just before serving. Reduce the heat and let simmer for 45 to 60 minutes. Serves 3-4

## Banana Cream Pie

| 4 c. nut milk | ¹/₄ t. salt |
| ¹/₂ c. unsweetened coconut, opt. | 1 t. vanilla |
| ¹/₂ c. starch | 4 ripe bananas |

Put the first five ingredients in a saucepan. Cook, stirring constantly until thick. Mash two bananas and add to mixture. Do not cook bananas. Slice the other bananas and add. Pour into Pie Crust and chill until set. May use Granola for crust and topping, making individual servings in custard cups. Serves 6-8.

## Pie Crust

Moisten pie pan with water. Sprinkle a ¹/₄ inch layer of wheat germ onto it. Fill with banana cream or other filling. Variations: nut meal, bread crumbs or dry cereal flakes, granola or granola meal made by blenderizing granola.

## Granola

| 12 c. oats | 1 T. salt |
| 3 apples, peeled, chopped small | 1 T. vanilla |
| 3-4 c. applesauce | |

Mix ingredients lightly together. Use a little water if needed. The more water used, the harder will be the finished product. Spread out in pans and bake at 275 degrees until entirely dry and lightly browned. Stir occasionally.

## Stewed Apricots

Cover dried apricots with water and let soak several hours, or until sufficient water has been absorbed to make them soft. Simmer slowly until thoroughly softened. Thicken the water with a little corn starch or arrowroot. 1 teaspoon of thickener stirred in 2-3 tablespoons of cold water needs to be added for each cupful of stewing apricots. Serve with oat waffles.

## Cantaloupe Sherbet

Peel very ripe cantaloupes, remove seeds and blend lightly to a liquid. Freeze. When ready to serve, chop into small chunks with a cleaver or ice pick. Blend alone or with a small amount of nut milk. May be put through a Champion Juicer. This is very good for diabetics because of its high content of myo-inositol.

## Vanilla Ice Cream

1 c. cashews
1 t. Slippery Elm powder (optional, but makes it creamy)
1 T. vanilla
$^1/_4$ t. salt

3 c. water-fresh fruit (peaches, blueberries, etc) may be substituted for part of the water

Blend all ingredients and freeze in ice cube trays or thin sheets. Follow the directions for the preceding "Ice Cream" recipe when you are ready to serve it. Slippery Elm powder gives a smooth, creamy texture.

## Ice Cream

1 c. ground, blanched almonds
1 can coconut milk (14 oz.), or 1 $^3/_4$ c. double-strength soymilk or nut milk
$^1/_2$ c. pineapple concentrate, plus a little more for blending
pinch of salt

4 c. water
$^1/_2$ c. apple concentrate
2 T. vegetable gelatin melted in $^1/_4$ c. water
1 T. vanilla

Whirl all ingredients in blender until smooth. Freeze in ice cube trays or thin sheets for easy handling. At serving time, put through a Champion Juicer or thaw until barely beginning to melt and whirl in blender, adding a bit of pineapple juice or fresh banana to make blender blades turn. Should have the consistency of soft ice cream.

## Easy Banana Ice Cream

Take skins off several very ripe bananas and freeze bananas. When ready to serve, put through a Champion Juicer or let thaw a tiny bit and whirl in blender. If needed, add a bit of fruit juice to bananas to turn blender.

## Banana Ice Cream II

2 ripe bananas
4 oz. soy milk
½ T. vanilla extract (optional)
4 raw pecans (optional)
   Peel, freeze, then defrost bananas 3-5 minutes. Slice into ½ to 1 inch slices, blenderize with milk and nuts. Variations: Use other natural fruits or nuts - peaches, strawberries or blueberries, any unsweetened jams.


## Frutari

2 c. crushed pineapple
12 oz. frozen apple or orange juice concentrate
3 T. Emes Gelatin
¼ c. chopped dates
1 c. pineapple juice

Mix, freeze, put through a Champion Juicer or blenderize. Delightful!


## Tofutari

2 t. Emes Gelatin
⅓ c. water
1 c. dates
1 lb. soft tofu, drained (2 c.)
1 ½ c. nut or soy milk
⅓ c. well cooked rice or spaghetti
2 t. vanilla or other flavors, nuts or coconut

   Soften gelatin by 3 minutes of soaking followed by heating to a boil. Blend all ingredients, freeze, put through a Champion Juicer, or blenderize.

## Carob Fudge Balls

Finely grind in electric food mill:
   5 t. sunflower seeds
   5 t. pumpkin seeds

Mix with:
    2 t. macaroon coconut
    5 t. carob powder
    ½ c. chopped pecans
    ½ c. chopped raisins
    ½ c. chopped dates
    2-3 t. water

Make ¾ inch balls and roll in unsweetened macaroon coconut. Note: much easier to form balls if mixture is refrigerated first.
Makes about 30 balls.

## *Meal Planner*

The meal planner that follows is helpful when you are beginning to learn how to prepare balanced meals with your new Health Recovery Diet. Each breakfast and lunch contains enough varieties of food to insure intake of the proper amounts of nutrients.

## Meal Planner

| | Main Dish | Second Dish | Raw Dish | Whole Grain Bread | Spreads, Nuts, Olives or Avocado |
|---|---|---|---|---|---|
| *Sunday* | | | | | |
| Breakfast | Fruited Oats | | Blackberry Sauce | Corn Bread | pumpkin seed (1 oz.) |
| Dinner | Potato Souffle | Asparagus | carrot strips | Whole Wheat Bread | olives (4-6) |
| *Monday* | | | | | |
| Breakfast | Baked Grits Squares | Pear Butter | grapes | Whole Wheat Toast | Cashew Gravy |
| Dinner | Chop Suey | Brown Rice | Cole Slaw | Soy Crackers | Soy Sour Cream |
| *Tuesday* | | | | | |
| Breakfast | Buckwheat-Rice Cereal | Stewed Apricots | orange | Melba Toast | Almond Milk |
| Dinner | Corn Tamale Pie | English Peas | sliced tomatoes | Hush Puppies | Gravy |
| *Wednesday* | | | | | |
| Breakfast | Corn Meal Soufflé | Sautéed Apples | pear | Oatmeal Thins | Soyonnaise II |
| Dinner | Shephard Pie | | onion slices | Whole Wheat Bread | |
| *Thursday* | | | | | |
| Breakfast | Oat Waffles | Stewed Apricots | plums (2) | Carrot Corn Bread | Emulsified Peanut Btr |
| Dinner | Lentils | Cabbage | shredded carrots | | olives (4-6) |
| *Friday* | | | | | |
| Breakfast | Corn Meal Mush | Apple Dumplings | orange | Melba Toast | Soyonnaise |
| Dinner | Oat Burgers | sliced tomatoes/onions | Alfalfa Sprouts | Burger Buns | Mustard & Catsup |
| *Sabbath* | | | | | |
| Breakfast | Auf Lauf | Thickened Fruit Juice | peaches | Corn Bread | Nut Milk |
| Dinner | Tofu, Oven Method | Zuccini Squash | lettuce wedges | Melba Toast | Gravy |

## Meal Planner

| | Main Dish | Second Dish | Raw Dish | Whole Grain Bread | Spreads, Nuts, Olives or Avocado |
|---|---|---|---|---|---|
| *Sunday* | | | | | |
| Breakfast | **Oatmeal** | | **Fruit Sauce** | Melba Toast | Peanut Butter |
| Dinner | Spanish Rice | | sliced tomatoes | Corn Dodgers | olives (4-6) |
| *Monday* | | | | | |
| Breakfast | **Rice Pudding** | Stewed Baked Pears | seedless grapes | Sesame Straws | Nut Milk |
| Dinner | Dry Beans | Summer Squash | celery sticks | Yeast Biscuits | Peanut Butter |
| *Tuesday* | | | | | |
| Breakfast | **French Toast** | Applesauce or strawberries | tart apple | | Pecan Butter |
| Dinner | Dry Rice | Bean Soup | carrot strips | Wheat Sticks | avocado |
| *Wednesday* | | | | | |
| Breakfast | **Millet** | | **Fruit Sauce** | Melba Toast | **Emulsified Peanut Butter** |
| Dinner | Split Pea Soup | Butternut Squash | **Cucumber/Lemon Juice** | Croutons | pumpkin seed (1 oz.) |
| *Thursday* | | | | | |
| Breakfast | **Baked Oatmeal** | **Stewed Peaches** | blackberries | Popcorn | **Carob-Nut Milk** |
| Dinner | Garbanzos | Corn & Okra | lettuce | Baked Corn | olives (4-6) |
| *Friday* | | | | | |
| Breakfast | **Granola** | Fruit Sauce | cherries | Rye Toast | **Sesame Butter** |
| Dinner | "Salmon Loaf" | Zucchini Gumbo | tomato | Oat Buns | Gravy |
| *Sabbath* | | | | | |
| Breakfast | **Grits** | | apples | Melba Toast | **Soyonnaise II** |
| Dinner | Bean Puree over split Corn Muffins | Brussel Spouts | bell peppers | Corn Muffins | French Dressing |

**Bold Print Indicates Recipe Names**

# CHAPTER TWELVE

# *Herbal Remedies Useful to Diabetics*

## *Herbal Teas*

The control of diabetes and hypoglycemia also includes the use of herbal remedies. Many varieties of herbs have proven useful in primitive societies for different conditions. The benefits of these herbs have only recently been studied by Western physicians and researchers, who are now prescribing them more frequently. The following list includes herbs which have been found to have a beneficial effect in the treatment of diabetes and hypoglycemia:

## *Herbs for Blood Sugar*

*Blueberry.* The root, bark and leaf have all been used. The root and bark must be simmered, but leaves only steeped. Prepare a decoction by putting one tablespoon of the root or bark in a quart of water and boil gently for $1/2$ hour. Prepare an infusion by pouring one quart of boiling water over one heaping tablespoon of the leaves. Do not boil. Let it steep for 30 minutes. Make these teas fresh daily; herbs lose much of their potency after 24 hours. Store them in the refrigerator during the day. Drink one cup, four times a day.

*Garlic.* One to two cloves with each meal has been used for generations to prevent and treat cancer, treat infections and to bring blood pressure down. It also has a specific ingredient for decreasing blood sugar levels.

*Fenugreek Seed.* Fenugreek seeds have been shown to lower glucose, cholesterol and triglyceride levels in the blood. Grind one half cup of seeds in a seed grinder (often sold as small coffee bean grinders). Sprinkle half of the ground seeds on each meal daily. Grind fresh daily and store in the refrigerator.

Other herbs that have been used for diabetes include Mistletoe, Bean Pods, Guggul, Walnut, Swedish Bitters, Bay Leaf, Oregano, Sage, Dandelion Leaf, and others which you may find in any good herb book.

### Herbs For Pain

Herbs have also been used effectively for reducing and eliminating pain. They are less expensive than drugs and rarely have side effects. When using most herbs you can feel secure knowing that no new problems will develop which are caused by the medicine, as so often happens with drugs. Another advantage with herbs is they are not addicting. They work in a nutritive and not a toxic way as do drugs. The following is an effective herbal pain formula:

| | |
|---|---|
| White Willow Bark | Black Cohosh |
| Blue Cohosh | Wild Lettuce |
| Skullcap | St. John's Wort |

Boil one quart of water. Turn flame down to a gentle boil. Add one teaspoon each of White Willow Bark and Black Cohosh. Simmer for 25 minutes. Turn flame off and add one teaspoon each of Blue Cohosh, Wild Lettuce, Skullcap and St. John's Wort. Cover and steep for 25 minutes. Take half a cup to one cup as needed for pain. If you take more than 1 and 1/2 to 2 quarts per day, you might get a mild headache from the Black Cohosh. If this happens, simply omit it from the mixture when you make your next batch.

## Sedative Herbs

Catnip                  Scullcap

Hops                    Valerian Root

Mint

Prepare the Valerian Root by boiling one quart of water. Turn flame down to a gentle boil, add one tablespoon of the root and simmer for 30 minutes. Valerian has been known to have a stimulating instead of a sedative effect for some people. If you find yourself stimulated after drinking Valerian, rather than relaxed, use the other herbs listed.

To prepare Catnip, Hops, Mint and Skullcap, pour one quart of boiling water (or the simmered Valerian Root tea if you wish to mix several herbs or try them all. Mix with the Valerian tea right after it has simmered) over one tablespoon of any or all of these herbs. Stir and steep for 25 minutes. Sometimes, using a combination of herbs is more effective than using one herb alone.

## Antibiotic Herbs

*Garlic.* Use 1-5 cloves, or 1-2 teaspoons of powder, or 2-4 capsules or 6-8 tablets of Kyolic as one dose. For very serious infections, take a dose
every 3-4 hours around the clock, setting clock at night. When improvement is noted, drop back to every 5-6 hours and finally 4 times daily for 5 days after all signs of infection have gone.

*Goldenseal, Echinacea and Chaparral.* Prepare the Goldenseal and Echinacea as you would the Valerian Root (under sedative herbs). Add one tablespoon of each to one quart of water. After they have simmered for 30 minutes, add one tablespoon of the Chaparral and let steep for 25 minutes. Take a cupful every 1-2 hours around the clock until improvements are observed, then cut down to every 4 hours in the daytime only. Continue tea for 5 days after all signs of infection have cleared.

### Diuretic Teas

*Dandelion.* Leaves or roots may be used. Fresh leaves may be added to a salad. A small handful will be effective to cause diuresis. If dried leaves are used, put 1/2 ounce (about 2 heaping teaspoons) per cup of boiling water. Steep 10-20 minutes. Use three to six cups daily. If dried roots are used, gently boil 2 to 3 teaspoons of powdered root per cup of water for 15 minutes. Use three to six cups daily. If you have the tincture, use 1 to 2 teaspoons, three to six times daily.

*Buchu.* Use 1 to 2 teaspoons dried leaves per cup of boiling water. Steep 10 to 20 minutes. Drink three to six cups daily.

*Uva Ursi.* Use one teaspoon per cup of boiling water. Steep 20 to 30 minutes. Use three to six cups per day. May turn the urine green. If the tannins in Uva Ursi cause nausea, you may use a teaspoon of unsweetened soy milk powder in each cup of tea, which should eliminate the problem.

*Corn Silk* and ground *Watermelon Seed* are also diuretic. Make teas in the same way Uva Ursi tea is made.

## Herbal Remedies For Foot Soaking for Fungus Disease or Other Foot Problems

1. Goldenseal, Thyme, Garlic, Witch Hazel and Comfrey Root can be used to make water solutions. Boil one cup of water, turn flame off and add one tablespoon of an herb. Steep for 30 minutes and add to the warm foot bath. Be cautious not to let the water for the foot bath become hotter than 103-104 degrees for the diabetic. 99-102 degrees is safer for the diabetic.
2. For an alcohol-herbal preparation: Use four ounces of any herb listed above to one pint of alcohol. Let soak for two weeks and shake twice daily. At the

end of two weeks, strain and store the liquid. Add one tablespoon to each quart of warm water.

3. One clove of garlic can be blended in one to two quarts of water and used as a solution to bathe the feet, or it may be applied after showering or used as an application during the day.

4. If walking is difficult, a poultice of red clover tea may be useful. Boil a cup of water, turn off the heat and add one tablespoon of tea. Let it steep for 20 minutes. Pour some of this onto a clean, cotton cloth and wrap around the affected areas of your feet. Leave on for one to six hours. Never put your shoes on if oily ointments or moist poultices are being used, because the skin of the feet will become soft and cause blisters where the shoes rub when you walk. Also, the likelihood of getting a severe inflammation is increased.

# *Epilogue*

The study of diabetes and hypoglycemia is a continuing work. We are grateful to acknowledge the present contributions of researchers working in the fields of diet and lifestyle as these relate to many of our contemporary diseases. Without the knowledge gained from these, and our own studies and experiences, the positive message of this book could never have been presented.

We hope you will benefit from the facts introduced throughout these pages. We also hope that if you, or someone you know is suffering with diabetes or hypoglycemia, you will apply these principles and see for yourself how the health of a friend or loved one (or your own health) will improve. You have nothing to lose by trying, and everything to gain by achieving a more satisfying quality of life.

*"Beloved, I wish above all things that thou mayest prosper and be in health, even as thy soul prospereth." III John 2.*

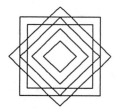

# *Appendix*

## *Interesting or Important Features About Blood Sugar Disease*

1. *The Process is Gradual:* People do not suddenly change from being healthy to being ill with diabetes. They often go through a phase of hypoglycemia with its general symptoms of fatigue and headache, its nervous system symptoms of depression and mental inefficiency and various digestive system problems. Both diabetes and hypoglycemia are part of the same syndrome. One comes at the beginning and the other towards the end of the degenerative process.

2. *Early Maturation a Cause:* As we noted in Chapter Two, Dr. Otto Schaefer, who worked with the Eskimos, argued that early menarche is due to a diet of store-bought foods, particularly a diet that includes the use of sugar and sugar products, as compared to later menarche with home grown, non-sugary food. This shift in diet brings on hypoglycemia and diabetes, and as we saw in the Eskimos it also causes acne, obesity, gallbladder disease, atherosclerosis, tooth decay, appendicitis and tonsillitis. Sugar and fat combined, especially when eaten along with generous amounts of dairy products and meat, appeared to Dr. Schaefer to be the destructive elements.

3. *Hypoglycemia Develops With Age:* Reactive or functional hypoglycemia is present to some degree in 70% of the adult population, whereas it is rare in children.

4. *Incidence Increases:* Since 1960 the incidence of diabetes has doubled in Austria, Italy, Switzerland and Venezuela, and almost tripled in Japan. The in-

cidence of hypoglycemia follows the same pattern.

5. *A Total Nutrient Disorder:* If we blamed all the symptoms of the hypoglycemic syndrome on a low sugar level, it would be the same as saying that one was ill with typhoid because of headache and diarrhea. These are symptoms of typhoid but there is much more to typhoid than these symptoms. It is simplistic to explain or treat typhoid in this way, and the same is true for hypoglycemia.

Hypoglycemia includes problems with salt and water balance (most patients are chronically dehydrated), weight control, autonomic nervous system overstimulation, signs of low oxygen in the central nervous system and malnutrition.

Dr. Demetrio Sodi-Pallares, a Mexican cardiologist, teaches that excessive intake of sodium in the form of salt, baking soda, baking powder, certain drugs containing sodium compounds and other forms of sodium, interfere with the proper function of the beta cells of the pancreas, and are factors in the genesis of diabetes.

6. *Magnesium, Manganese, Chromium and Vanadium Important:* The physiological importance of magnesium is becoming more apparent. A recent discovery highlights the fact that insulin and other hormones may function by binding or releasing magnesium within the cells. Deficiencies are quite common.

Magnesium is known to be an activator of enzymes and necessary for the normal regulation of body temperature, synthesis of protein, contraction of muscles and transmission of nerve impulses. A deficiency of a related element, manganese, has also been associated with impaired glucose tolerance. Whole grains, nuts, dry beans and leafy green vegetables are good sources of magnesium and manganese.

Chromium is essential to a host of vital processes including carbohydrate metabolism. It is deficient in the average, refined American diet. Older people suffer more severely from chromium deficiency than younger people. The chromium levels in older Americans are drastically lower than the levels in comparable age groups in countries such as the Middle and Far East, and many nations of Africa.

Impaired glucose tolerance is the hallmark of chromium deficiency. Using chromium levels in hair as a measure, a dropoff in chromium was found after the first few months of life in those who developed impaired glucose tolerance. An even more abrupt decrease was found in women after giving birth. Chromium levels can be enhanced by eating Brewer's yeast.

Dr. John Scharffenberg, a physician/nutritionist who was involved in research at Loma Linda University, has reported exciting findings about the trace mineral, vanadium. In animals made experimentally diabetic, vanadium brought the blood sugar to normal. Researchers are trying to incorporate vanadium into an organic form, so it will be absorbed better by the body. Vanadium can then be given to patients in supplemental doses larger than the natural amounts which occur in foods. Foods in which there is a high content of vanadium are listed in Chapter Eleven.

7. *Protein Not Always a Friend:* Excess proteins may be greater villains than was once thought, because of their role in producing hardening of the arteries, liver and kidney disease and an increased cancer risk. In the United States, diabetics and hypoglycemics have traditionally been given a high-protein, high-fat diet. The hypoglycemic syndrome can be expected to be aggravated by a high protein diet in some patients. This aggravation may be due to an enhanced insulinotropic (attracted to insulin) effect of amino acids. A low protein content should be a feature in a regular diet as well as in a diabetic or hypoglycemic diet.

Four groups of rabbits were tested; one on a normal diet, a second on a high cholesterol diet, a third on a high protein diet and a fourth on a combined high cholesterol and high protein diet. Those on the last diet had the greatest amount of atherosclerosis.[82]

8. *What Causes the Blood Sugar Rise?:* Within five minutes after food reaches the stomach there is a considerable rise in both glucose and insulin in the blood, particularly insulin. The levels continue to rise until they reach a peak, 30-45 minutes later. Blood sugar rises slowly after a high fiber meal, but it rises quickly after eating refined, low fiber foods. Several gastrointestinal enzymes begin to be produced at the onset of a meal and these also stimulate the secretion of insulin. All of these represent major changes occurring at the same time one is eating, but they do not happen when one is fasting. When we eat a sugary, fatty or refined snack, it encourages increased production of stress hormones, digestive enzymes and insulin. These processes begin immediately and cause the body to put forth a huge energy expenditure.

9. *Symptoms Related to Highs and Lows in Sugar:* Low blood sugar after meals produces symptoms in the autonomic nervous system between one and five hours after meals. The faster this fall occurs after the high swing of sugar upward following refined carbohydrate meals, the more prominent the symptoms. Most people with a blood sugar level below 55 will show symptoms and many will do so below 65.
Sometimes a patient's history will include many symptoms specific for this syndrome, even though the laboratory has not shown low blood sugar yet. This means the body is making a herculean effort to keep all the mechanisms healthy, but stress on these mechanisms is causing symptoms.

When the blood sugar drops too low, certain alarm bells go off in the body and several emergency actions are triggered. First, the adrenal glands are stimulated to release catecholamines, which are comprised of adrenalin (also called epinephrine) or norepinephrine. Increased cortisol and steroid hormones are produced. The adrenalin speeds to the liver and muscles and begins to break down the glycogen which is stored there. Adrenalin converts the glycogen into glucose in order to raise the blood sugar back up to normal. Extra insulin is secreted from the pancreas in an attempt to establish the normal sugar balance in the blood. The effects of the extra adrenalin and insulin cause symptoms that are quite distressing. The heart begins to race, the blood pressure goes up, there is nervousness, a jittery feeling and dizziness.

If the heart racing rises to 100-150 beats per minute, it will stimulate the sympathetic nervous system. This is part of the "fight or flight" response, and was designed for protection when a dangerous circumstance threatens. But for a person experiencing hypoglycemic reactions, there is no menacing occurrence forcing him or her into fighting or running. These reactions are the result of strain from all the strong chemical reactions going on in the body. These patients are usually sitting down with pounding hearts, feeling ill, uncomfortable and confused.

The stimulation of the sympathetic nervous system also causes the blood sugar to rise. It raises the cholesterol and triglyceride levels in the blood as well. These fatty substances, along with the catecholamines, can increase the stickiness or sludginess of the platelets in the blood, which adds to the risk of clotting and impaired circulation.

Stressful situations, even imagining stressful situations, will stimulate various centers, such as the hypothalamus in the brain. This in turn stimulates the pituitary gland, which activates the central nervous system and the pancreas. Hypoglycemic symptoms are mainly due to nervous system mechanisms responding to stress. These symptoms may take the form of the "flight" response and be expressed as running away from certain responsibilities in life.

People who have been labelled neurotic may be chronically under- responsive in the glucose tolerance test. Their symptoms include paranoia, strange thoughts and depression. These symptoms usually occur when hypoglycemia has become a chronic condition. A typical history for these patients includes fatigue, allergies, insomnia, frequent upper respiratory tract infections (many of which were treated with antibiotics which add another strain), blackouts, poor concentration, dermatitis, hives, scant perspiration, no thirst which results in chronic dehydration, craving for salt, eating too many sweets and fermented foods like cheese and vinegar, eating too many salty foods such as nuts and chips, rapid growth during the ages of five to ten years, palpitations and many other expressions of allergies.

10. *"Average" Laboratory Levels Not "Normal"*: Average is often wrongly termed normal in regard to carbohydrate levels. The accepted normals are usually too broad. Most people who have blood sugar levels in the 60's, or even in the 50's, will experience improvement or disappearance of some symptoms once they begin a proper health program. We may never know whether it was the diet, the exercise or the regularity that brought about the change, because these are all equally important.

Flat glucose tolerance curves do not usually produce anxiety attacks, as compared to the reactive curves which are characteristically associated with anxiety. Avoid refined carbohydrates! They may trigger a hypoglycemic reaction and stress.

## Laboratory Values, both Ideal and Average Reference Range

| Chemistry Report | Ideal Range | Average Range |
|---|---|---|
| Glucose | 70-85 | 60-115 |
| Blood Urea Nitrogen | 4-15 | 6-23 |
| Sodium | 134-140 | 135-145 |
| Iron | 30-100 | 40-150 |
| Uric Acid | 1-5 | 2-8 |
| Cholesterol | 100 plus your age | 120-200 |
| Triglycerides | Below 100 | 30-175 |

| **Complete Blood Count** | | |
|---|---|---|
| White Blood Cells | 3.0-5.5 | 4.8-10.8 |
| | *Women at sea level* | |
| Red Blood Cells | *3.0-4.0* | *4.2-5.4* |
| | Men at sea level | |
| | 4.2-5.0 | 4.7-6.1 |
| | *Women at sea level* | |
| Hemoglobin | *10.5-12.5* | *12-16* |
| | Men at sea level | |
| | 12.0-14.5 | 14-18 |
| | *Women at sea level* | |
| Hematocrit | *31.5-37.5* | *37-47* |
| | Men at sea level | |
| | 35-43.5 | 42-52 |

11.  *Glucagon:* Glucagon is involved with the movement of fats, the secretion of insulin and glucose need. Every organ system in the body is involved in producing glucagon. Even the intestinal mucosa secretes a glucagon-like material. Glucagon stimulates the release of catecholamine, which is part of the stress hormone group. Glucagon may be the first hormone to begin acting in the embryo. The cells producing glucagon appear earlier in the pancreas of embryonic rats than the insulin-producing cells. Glucagon is 100 times more active in the first secretions of the pancreas than insulin.

Glucagon also participates in causing elevated blood sugars. Diabetics have 2-3 times greater glucagon responses than normal people. Excessive glucagon secretion is partly responsible for high blood sugar levels after meals.

When there is a reduction in blood sugar, glucagon rises in the normal person, followed by a rise in glucose. This helps us to function without food for extended periods. A healthy person should be able to fast for several days and experience no disability and no discomfort except hunger. An insulin-dependent diabetic should never fast. If insulin is not taken, the fast will bring on acidosis and ketoacidosis. Non-insulin-dependent diabetics may be experience significant health benefits by fasting for one to two days per week.

The relative insulin:glucagon level is more important than the absolute level of either one alone. Insulin is responsible for keeping the blood sugar from going too high and glucagon from going too low. The body is designed to function at its optimum level when these two hormones maintain a proper relationship.

When something happens to the insulin:glucagon mechanism and the proper proportions of insulin and glucagon cannot be maintained, profound changes occur in metabolism. Amino acids are the most precious material controlled by this ratio. Glycolysis (the breakdown of glucose to form energy) and gluconeogenesis (making glucose from proteins, etc.) which are nearly equally important processes, will not function properly if the insulin/glucagon mechanism is off balance.[83] An appropriate pancreatic response by the body to fasting, eating and other demands for insulin and glucagon, may spell the difference between health and disease.

12. *Brain Uses Glucose:* Many tissues, such as the brain, are utterly dependent on glucose for fuel. Nerve tis

sues also make energy using only glucose, while all other tissues use protein and fat for energy as well. If the brain does not have enough glucose, such as when the blood sugar level drops too low, symptoms such as a foggy-brain, dizziness and weakness begin to show up. Clear thinking becomes a problem and there is the potential for blackouts. Alcohol and the hypoglycemia associated with it will destroy brain cells, produce convulsions and even cause death.

13. *Somatostatin:* Somatostatin has been found in the hypothalamus, the pancreas and small intestine. Somatostatin suppresses growth hormone, affects platelet aggregation (having to do with blood clotting), lowers glucagon levels and inhibits gastrin, a stomach hormone which stimulates gastric secretions. Overproduction of glucagon may be prevented by somatostatin. Glucagon levels rise in response to the production of adrenal hormones which are manufactured during stress.

14. *Growth Hormone Produced More:* Growth hormone increases with diabetes and the hypoglycemic syndrome. Normally, the level of growth hormone rises very slightly after meals, during times of emotional tension, with exercise and general activity. In the diabetic child there are more peaks of growth hormone during the day. This results in a larger body size. In the child this is seen as accelerated growth and in the adult as obesity.

15. *Stomach Sluggishness Causes Some Cases of Hypoglycemia:* The flat curve hypoglycemic may represent a missed high blood sugar phase which occurred faster than 30 minutes in the first blood specimen drawn after a test meal. The flat curve may also be due to retention of food in the stomach.

16. *Pregnancy and Slow Stomach Emptying May Cause Some Symptoms:* Gastric emptying time is slightly slower in pregnant women than in women who are

not pregnant and intestinal absorption of glucose is enhanced.

17. *Hypoglycemia and Gastric Surgery:* Hypoglycemia may be the result of surgical removal of part of the stomach. Dumping after meals then occurs and sugar literally explodes into the bloodstream.

18. *Drugs and Chemicals Multiply Problems:* Many common drugs cause derangements in blood glucose; alcohol, salicylates, oral contraceptives, diuretics, cardiac drugs, steroids, Dilantin and Levodopa.

19. *Beverage Alcohol and Hypoglycemia:* Beverage alcohol causes hypoglycemia because it temporarily destroys the ability of the liver to engage in gluconeogenesis. Alcohol may also act on insulin secretion through a permanent metabolic change in the beta cells of the pancreas. Life-threatening hypoglycemia has been known to result from small amounts of alcohol taken in a fasting state. Alcohol is by far the commonest cause of profound, disabling and lethal hypoglycemic coma in diabetic children and adults alike. Children may become comatose an hour after they have drunk what is left in cocktail glasses at a party.

20. *Stress:* The hyperglycemia (high blood sugar) of stress may be more related to the pancreatic hormone, glucagon, than to release of sugar by the liver. A sudden loud noise causes a four-fold rise in plasma glucagon levels. The blood glucose level may rise 25%. In experiments with animals, the injection of endotoxin (from bacteria) causes a similar rise in glucagon, but no change in glucose.

The functionally diabetic state can be produced in anyone by stress. This is probably the commonest form of acute elevation of blood sugar. The cooperation between insulin and glucagon is very sensitive and maintains blood sugar within a very narrow range, perhaps 10 mg. during most of the day, with the exception of the time immediately after eating. Many borderline diabetics will have sugar in the urine during a period of stress. If immediate preventive measures are not taken, most of these borderline cases will eventually become full-blown diabetics. Stress can come from injury, surgery, disease of any kind, pregnancy, overweight and even overeating.

21. *City Living Causes Stress:* Illustrating how the noise, the overcrowding and the activity of city life makes a change in biology, it has been observed that urban cats are darker than country cats, which is a result of excessive adrenal activity. Physical reactions to stress happen to human populations as well as to the pet populations that share the same environment.

22. *Cow's Milk:* The hypoglycemic activity of cow's milk is felt to be due to a high level of the amino acid leucine, which stimulates insulin to be more active. Cow's milk should be avoided by hypoglycemics because of its amino acid and sugar content, both of which are harmful to human metabolism. It should also be avoided by overweight people because the insulin produced in response to leucine can cause the appetite to increase. Human milk has a lower content of casein and less hypoglycemic activity.

23. *Enormous Sugar Use:* More than 7-8% of individuals in the United States are diabetic. Approximately 50% of the carbohydrates consumed in the United States are in the form of refined sugars. The refined sugar habit is begun at birth in the hospital with sugar water and artificial formulas. This is a faulty and dangerous practice and could be a factor in the development of insulin resistance. Many people develop hypoglycemia when eating simple sugars such as table sugar, honey, malt and syrups with a meal. This happens especially with the development of excessive hunger after self-imposed

carbohydrate restriction [84] or drinking alcohol with a meal.

Most hypoglycemics have discovered that if they eat or drink something sweet, their symptoms will disappear. The sweet food or drink raises the blood sugar and makes the person feel better for a short time. But this is a yo-yo process which needs to be repeated when the blood sugar falls again and leads to increased sugar consumption in a person who is usually already eating too much sugar.

We are not able to handle more than three to five teaspoons of sugar in one day without suffering physical damage. For many people, physical injury may happen with an even smaller amount of sugar. Yet, the average soft drink contains almost one teaspoon of sugar per ounce!

24. *Fruit Juice Promotes Hypoglycemia:* Ten normal subjects were given test meals of 60 grams of carbohydrates in the form of various types of apples. 17 minutes were required to ingest the apples, six minutes for the puree, and one and a-half minutes for the juice. When the three meals were eaten at the same time, the resulting satiety assessed on a 20 point scale was significantly greater with the apples than with the puree, and the puree was rated over the juice. Fiber slows carbohydrate digestion, induces satisfaction and prevents rebound hypoglycemia, presumably by moderating insulin secretion. The blood sugar rose to similar levels after all three meals. However, there was a striking fall in blood sugar with the juice, a less striking fall with the puree and the rapid fall was not seen with whole apples.[85] [86] We can conclude, as a general rule, it is more healthful to eat whole fruits than either purees or juices.

25. *Begin at Birth for Prevention:* Many types of neurologic symptoms such as fast heart rate, sweating, tremulousness, confusion and coma may be produced

by low blood sugar. Curtailing refined sugars to less than five percent of the carbohydrate intake, starting at birth, should keep diabetes from appearing. This would mean limiting sugar intake to two teaspoons or less per day.

## BOOKS RECOMMENDED

*HOME REMEDIES*: **HYDROTHERAPY, MASSAGE, CHARCOAL, AND OTHER SIMPLE TREATMENTS,** Agatha Moody Thrash, M.D., and Calvin L. Thrash, Jr., M.D., NewLifestyle Books, 30 Uchee Pines Rd., Ste.15, Seale, AL 36875, 1982 [79]

*NUTRITION FOR VEGETARIANS* , Agatha Moody Thrash, M.D., and Calvin L. Thrash, Jr., M.D., NewLifestyle Books, 30 Uchee Pines Rd., Ste.15, Seale, AL 36875, 1981 [80]

*EAT FOR STRENGTH COOKBOOK,* both Regular and Oil-free editions by Agatha Moody Thrash, M.D., NewLifestyle Books, 30 Uchee Pines Rd. Ste. 15, Seale, AL 36875, 1978 [81]

# Bibliography

[1]  **Early Exposure to Cow's Milk and Solid Foods in Infancy.** *Diabetes*, 42:288, February, 1993

[2]  Donsbach, Kurt W., Ph.D., *What You Always Wanted to Know About Diabetes.* International Institute of Natural Health Sciences, 1981, p. 37-38

[3]  Diabetes Epidemiology Research International Group: Geographic Patterns of Childhood IDDM. *Diabetes*, 37:1113-1119, Aug. 1988

[4]  Tuomilehto, Jaakko, et al,**Coffee Consumption As Trigger For IDDM In Childhood.***British Medical Journal*, 300:642, March 10, 1990

[5]  **You Are What You Inherit.** *Nutrition Today*, 1986, 21:18-24

[6]  **Dietary Protein: A Trigger of Insulin-Dependent Diabetes in the BP Rat?** *Diabetologia*, 26:297-9, 1984

[7]  **Diabetes Epidemiology Research International Group: Geographic Patterns of Childhood IDDM.** *Diabetes*, 37:1113-1119. August, 1988

[8]  Lilleoja, Stephen et al. **Impaired GT as a Disorder of Insulin Action.** *New England Journal of Medicine*, 318:1217-1230, May 12, 1988

[9]  Polonsky, K.S. et al. **Abnormal Patterns of Insulin Secretion in NIDDM.** *New England Journal of Medicine*, 318:1231-1239

[10]  O'Rahilly, Stephen, et al. **Impaired Pulsatile Secretion of Insulin in Relatives of Patients with NIDDM.** *New England Journal of Medicine,* 318:1225-1230, May 12, 1988

[11]  *Nutrition Today*, May, 1987, p.43

[12]  *Diabetes Research*, 1991, 17:139-145

[13]  *Journal of Nutrition*, 1993, 123:626-623

[14]  *Journal of Clinical Medicine*, August, 1992, 33:1523-9

[15]  *Endocrinology*, February, 1993, 132:652, 646

[16]  *Journal of Clinical Endocrinology*, August, 1992, 37:2, pp. 147-155

[17] *Journal of Clinical Investigation*, July, 1992, 90:24-9

[18] Landsberg, Lewis, **The Insulin Resistance Syndrome.** *Focus on Hypertension*, January, 1993, p. 5

[19] Landsberg, Lewis, Harvard Medical School; **Insulin Resistance, Energy Balancing, and Sympathetic Nervous System Activity.** *Clinical and Experimental Hypertension, Part A, Theory and Practice*, Volume 12 Issue 5, 1990 p. 817-830

[20] *Journal of the American Medical Association*, January 6, 1993, 69:104

[21] *Archives of Internal Medicine*, February 8, 1993, 153:290

[22] *American Journal of Surgery*, January, 1993, 165:61

[23] *Diabetologia*, December, 1992, 35:1140

[24] *Science News*, September 16, 1989, 136:184-186

[25] Defronzo, Ralph, M.D., Professor of Medicine and Chief of Diabetes Section at the University of Texas, Health Science Center, San Antonio. Much of the information on insulin resistance came from a lecture delivered by Dr. DeFronzo at the University of Alabama at Birmingham in 1992.

[26] North, A Frederick Jr. et al. **A Secular Increase in the Incidence of Juvenile Diabetes Mellitus.** *Journal of Pediatrics*, Volume 91 No. 5, p. 706, November 1977

[27] *Diabetes Outlook*, July-August, 1978

[28] *Diabetes Outlook*, April-May, 1978

[29] *Diabetes Outlook*, April-May, 1978 p. 7

[30] Educational Reviews, Inc., Practical Reviews in Internal Medicine. Albert Einstein College of Medicine and Montefiore Medical Center. August, 1992

[31] North, A. Frederick Jr. et al. **Birth Weight, Gestational Age and Perinatal Deaths in 5,471 Infants of Diabetic Mothers.** *Journal of Pediatrics*, Volume 90 No. 3, p.444 March 1977

[32] Stehbens, J. A. et al. **Outcome at Ages One, Three and Five Years of Children Born to Diabetic Women.** *American Journal of Obstetrics and Gynecology*, 127:408, 1977

[33] *Internal Medicine News*, 1/1/78

[34] *Diabetes Outlook*, Sept. 1978 p.2

[35] *Family Practice News*, October 1, 1978 p.12

[36] Gunby, Phil. Viral Link Sought in Juvenile Diabetes. *Journal of the American Medical Association,* 240(12):1219, September 15, 1978

[37] *Diabetes Outlook,* April-May, 1978 p. 1

[38] Menser, Margaret et al. **Rubella Infections and Diabetes Mellitus.** *Lancet,* 1:57 January 14, 1978

[39] *Diabetes Outlook,* 12(5):1, May-June 1977

[40] *Physician's Desk Reference,* 1992 p. 1092

[41] *Diabetes Outlook,* February 1979 p. 2

[42] *Lancet,* October 15, 1977 p. 789

[43] *Diabetes Outlook,* 12(7):1, September, 1977

[44] *British Medical Journal,* 2:671, September 18, 1976

[45] *International Journal of the Indian Medical Association,* 57:201, September 16, 1971

[46] *Postgraduate Medicine,* February 1979, P. 23

[47] *MD,* 21:39 August, 1977

[48] Riccardi, G. et al. **Separate Influences of Dietary Carbohydrates and Fiber on Metabolic Control of Diabetes.** *Diabetologia,* 26:116-121, 1984

[49] *The Internist Reporter,* Aug. 1977, p. 23

[50] Brungell, John et al. **Effect of a Fat-Free, High Carbohydrate Diet on Diabetic Subjects With Fasting Hyperglycemia.** *Diabetes,* 23(2):138, February 1974

[51] *Modern Medicine,* May 30-June 15, 1978 p. 68

[52] Kent, Saul. **Reevaluating the Dietary Treatment of Diabetes.** *Geriatrics,* May 1978, p. 99

[53] Kiehm, Tae G., M.D. et al. **Beneficial Effects of a High Carbohydrate, High Fiber Diet on Hyperglycemic Diabetic Men.** *American Journal of Clinical Nutrition,* 29:898, August 1976

[54] Carpenter, Thorne M., Ph.D. et al. **The Utilization of Jerusalem Artichokes By A Patient With Diabetes.** *Archives of Internal Medicine,* 42:64 July 1928

[55] *Union Medical Du Canada,* 105:(8):1147-51, August, 1976

[56] Gupta, R.K. et al. **Blood Sugar Lowering Effect of Various Fractions of Onion.** *Indian Journal of Experimental Biology,* 13.01 15.313, April, 1977

[57] *Diabetes Outlook*, February 1979, p. 3

[58] *Internist Reporter*, 3:1, July 1977

[59] Turner, R.C. et al. **Changes in Plasma Insulin Ethanol-Induced Hypoglycemia.** *Metabolism*, Volume 22 Number 2 February 1973, p.111

[60] *Lancet*, 607, March 17, 1979

[61] Donsbach, Kurt, Ph.D., *What You Always Wanted to Know About Diabetes*, International Institute of Natural Health Sciences, 1981 p.35

[62] Ibid., p.38

[63] *Patient Care*, June 15, 1975 P.37

[64] *Today's Health*, July 1957

[65] *American Journal of Nursing*, May 1978, p. 888

[66] Duncan, Theodore G. M.D. **Teaching Commonsense Health Care Habits to Diabetic Patients.** *Geriatrics*, October 1976, p. 93

[67] *Eat For Strength Cookbook*, Agatha M. Thrash, M.D., FACP;    NewLifestyle Books, 1975

[68] Ibid.

[69] Ibid.

[70] **Exaggerated Hypoglycemia After a Pizza Meal in Well-Controlled Diabetes.** *Diabetes Care*, 16:678, 1993

[71] *Tohoku Journal of Experimental Medicine*, 140:411-412, 1980

[72] Rude, Robert, *Postgraduate Medicine*, 92:217-224, October, 1992

[73] Feinglos, Mark, M.D.; Duke University Professor of Diabetology. **Interview with Joe Graedon, published in People's Pharmacy,** *Albany Sunday Herald*, November 8, 1992

[74] *American Journal of Public Health*, February, 1993

[75] Batmanghelidj, F., M.D., *Your Body's Many Cries For Water*, Global Health, 1992

[76] *Patient Care*, April 30, 1991, p.45

[77] Baker, Elizabeth and Dr. Elton;*The Uncook Book*, Drelwood Publications, 1980, p. 183-186

[78] Ensminger, et. al.*Foods and Nutrition Encyclopedia*, 1983,

p.1234-1235
[79] *Home Remedies, Hydrotherapy, Massage, Charcoal and Other Simple Treatments;* Agatha Moody Thrash, M.D. and Calvin L. Thrash, Jr., M.D.; NewLifestyle Books, 30 Uchee Pines Rd., #15, Seale, AL 36875
[80] *Nutrition For Vegetarians,* Agatha Moody Thrash, M.D. and Calvin L. Thrash, Jr., M.D.; NewLifestyle Books, Seale, AL 36875
[81] *Eat For Strength*, Regular and Oil-Free Editions; Agatha Moody Thrash, M.D., NewLifestyle Books, Seale, AL 36875
[82] *Science News,* August 21, 1971
[83] Turner, R.C. et al. **Changes in Plasma Insulin Ethanol-Induced Hypoglycemia.** *Metabolism,* Volume 22 Number 2, February 1973 p. 111
[84] *Modern Medicine,* January 15-January 30, 1979, p. 49
[85] Haber, G.B. et al. **Depletion and Disruption of Dietary Fiber; Effects on Satiety, Glucose and Insulin.** *Lancet,* 2:679 October 1, 1977
[86] Heaton, K.W. et al. **How Fiber May Prevent Obesity: Promotion of Satiety and Prevention of Rebound Hypoglycemia.** *American Journal of Clinical Nutrition,* 31:S280, October 1978, Supplement

# *Index*

effect of fiber  70
minor increases injure  51, 52
Sympathetic nervous system  65

## T

Trust in divine power  160

## U

Urine sugar
errors in  47

## V

Viruses
Type I diabetes
may cause  75
Vitamin B$^{12}$  169
Viscosity, blood  77

## W

Weight, normal  156
Weight control  129
how to 151

# Uchee Pines...
## THE PLACE TO BE!

...for healing
...for rest
...for a new lifestyle

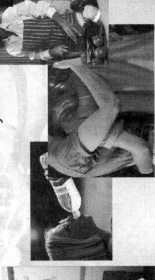

☐ YES, please send me more information about your natural treatment program.
☐ I'd like to talk with someone about the program. My number is ( ) _____

Name _____ Address _____

City _____ ST _____ Zip/Code _____ Country _____

Uchee Pines Lifestyle Center, 30 Uchee Pines Road, #75, Seale, AL 36875 USA 334/855-4764

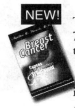
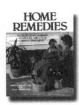
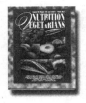